Integrating Health Care and Social Services for People with Serious Illness

PROCEEDINGS OF A WORKSHOP

Laurene Graig, Sylara Marie Cruz, and Joe Alper, *Rapporteurs*

Roundtable on Quality Care for People with Serious Illness

Board on Health Care Services

Board on Health Sciences Policy

Health and Medicine Division

The National Academies of
SCIENCES • ENGINEERING • MEDICINE

THE NATIONAL ACADEMIES PRESS
Washington, DC
www.nap.edu

THE NATIONAL ACADEMIES PRESS   500 Fifth Street, NW   Washington, DC 20001

This activity was supported by contract No. HHSN263201200074I (Task Order No. HHSN26300096) and by Aetna Inc., Altarum Institute, American Academy of Hospice and Palliative Medicine, American Cancer Society, American Geriatrics Society, Anthem, Inc., Ascension Health, Association of Professional Chaplains, Association of Rehabilitation Nurses, Blue Cross Blue Shield Association, Blue Cross Blue Shield of Massachusetts, Blue Cross and Blue Shield of North Carolina, Bristol-Myers Squibb, The California State University Institute for Palliative Care, Cambia Health Solutions, Cedars-Sinai Health System, Center to Advance Palliative Care, Centers for Medicare & Medicaid Services, Coalition to Transform Advanced Care, Common Practice, Excellus BlueCross BlueShield, Federation of American Hospitals, The Greenwall Foundation, The John A. Hartford Foundation, Hospice and Palliative Nurses Association, Kaiser Permanente, Susan G. Komen, Gordon and Betty Moore Foundation, National Coalition for Hospice and Palliative Care, National Hospice and Palliative Care Organization, National Institute of Nursing Research, National Palliative Care Research Center, National Patient Advocate Foundation, National Quality Forum, The New York Academy of Medicine, Oncology Nursing Society, Patient-Centered Outcomes Research Institute, Social Work Hospice and Palliative Care Network, Supportive Care Coalition, UnitedHealth Group, and the National Academy of Medicine. Any opinions, findings, conclusions, or recommendations expressed in this publication do not necessarily reflect the views of any organization or agency that provided support for the project.

International Standard Book Number-13: 978-0-309-48816-7
International Standard Book Number-10: 0-309-48816-8
Digital Object Identifier: https://doi.org/10.17226/25350

Additional copies of this publication are available from the National Academies Press, 500 Fifth Street, NW, Keck 100, Washington, DC 20001; (800) 624-6242 or (202) 334-3313; http://www.nap.edu.

Copyright 2019 by the National Academy of Sciences. All rights reserved.

Printed in the United States of America

Suggested citation: National Academies of Sciences, Engineering, and Medicine. 2019. *Integrating health care and social services for people with serious illness: Proceedings of a workshop*. Washington, DC: The National Academies Press. doi:10.17226/25350.

The National Academies of
SCIENCES · ENGINEERING · MEDICINE

The **National Academy of Sciences** was established in 1863 by an Act of Congress, signed by President Lincoln, as a private, nongovernmental institution to advise the nation on issues related to science and technology. Members are elected by their peers for outstanding contributions to research. Dr. Marcia McNutt is president.

The **National Academy of Engineering** was established in 1964 under the charter of the National Academy of Sciences to bring the practices of engineering to advising the nation. Members are elected by their peers for extraordinary contributions to engineering. Dr. C. D. Mote, Jr., is president.

The **National Academy of Medicine** (formerly the Institute of Medicine) was established in 1970 under the charter of the National Academy of Sciences to advise the nation on medical and health issues. Members are elected by their peers for distinguished contributions to medicine and health. Dr. Victor J. Dzau is president.

The three Academies work together as the **National Academies of Sciences, Engineering, and Medicine** to provide independent, objective analysis and advice to the nation and conduct other activities to solve complex problems and inform public policy decisions. The National Academies also encourage education and research, recognize outstanding contributions to knowledge, and increase public understanding in matters of science, engineering, and medicine.

Learn more about the National Academies of Sciences, Engineering, and Medicine at **www.nationalacademies.org**.

The National Academies of
SCIENCES · ENGINEERING · MEDICINE

Consensus Study Reports published by the National Academies of Sciences, Engineering, and Medicine document the evidence-based consensus on the study's statement of task by an authoring committee of experts. Reports typically include findings, conclusions, and recommendations based on information gathered by the committee and the committee's deliberations. Each report has been subjected to a rigorous and independent peer-review process and it represents the position of the National Academies on the statement of task.

Proceedings published by the National Academies of Sciences, Engineering, and Medicine chronicle the presentations and discussions at a workshop, symposium, or other event convened by the National Academies. The statements and opinions contained in proceedings are those of the participants and are not endorsed by other participants, the planning committee, or the National Academies.

For information about other products and activities of the National Academies, please visit www.nationalacademies.org/about/whatwedo.

PLANNING COMMITTEE FOR A WORKSHOP ON INTEGRATING HEALTH CARE AND SOCIAL SERVICES FOR PEOPLE WITH SERIOUS ILLNESS[1]

JOANNE LYNN (*Co-Chair*), Director, Center for Elder Care and Advanced Illness, Altarum Institute
JUDITH R. PERES (*Co-Chair*), Long-Term and Palliative Care Consultant, Clinical Social Worker and Board Member, Social Work Hospice and Palliative Care Network
ROBERT A. BERGAMINI, Medical Director, Palliative Care Services, Mercy Clinic Children's Cancer and Hematology, representing the Supportive Care Coalition
AMY J. BERMAN, Senior Program Officer, The John A. Hartford Foundation
HAIDEN HUSKAMP, 30th Anniversary Professor of Health Care Policy, Harvard Medical School
KIMBERLY JOHNSON, Associate Professor of Medicine, Senior Fellow in the Center for the Study of Aging and Human Development, Duke University School of Medicine
SUTEP LAOHAVANICH, Program Officer, Gordon and Betty Moore Foundation
JERI L. MILLER, Chief, Office of End-of-Life and Palliative Care Research and Senior Policy Analyst, Division of Extramural Science Programs, National Institute of Nursing Research, National Institutes of Health
SHARON SCRIBNER PEARCE, Vice President, Policy, National Hospice and Palliative Care Organization
JOANNE REIFSNYDER, Executive Vice President, Clinical Operations and Chief Nursing Officer, Genesis Healthcare, representing the Hospice and Palliative Nurses Association
KATRINA M. SCOTT, Oncology Chaplain, Massachusetts General Hospital, representing the Association of Professional Chaplains
JOSEPH W. SHEGA, Regional Medical Director, VITAS Hospice Care, representing the American Geriatrics Society

---

[1] The National Academies of Sciences, Engineering, and Medicine's planning committees are solely responsible for organizing the workshop, identifying topics, and choosing speakers. The responsibility for the published Proceedings of a Workshop rests with the workshop rapporteurs and the institution.

TANYA STEWART, Senior Medical Director, UnitedHealthcare Retiree Solutions

Project Staff

LAURENE GRAIG, Director, Roundtable on Quality Care for People with Serious Illness
SYLARA MARIE CRUZ, Research Assistant
RAJBIR KAUR, Senior Program Assistant
SHARYL NASS, Director, Board on Health Care Services, and Director, National Cancer Policy Forum
ANDREW M. POPE, Director, Board on Health Sciences Policy

Consultant

JOE ALPER, Consulting Writer

ROUNDTABLE ON QUALITY CARE FOR PEOPLE WITH SERIOUS ILLNESS[1]

LEONARD D. SCHAEFFER (*Chair*), Judge Robert Maclay Widney Chair and Professor, University of Southern California
JAMES A. TULSKY (*Vice Chair*), Chair, Department of Psychosocial Oncology and Palliative Care, Dana-Farber Cancer Institute; Chief, Division of Palliative Medicine, Brigham and Women's Hospital; Professor of Medicine and Co-Director, Center for Palliative Care, Harvard Medical School
JENNIFER BALLENTINE, Executive Director, The California State University Institute for Palliative Care
ROBERT A. BERGAMINI, Medical Director, Palliative Care Services, Mercy Clinic Children's Cancer and Hematology, representing the Supportive Care Coalition
AMY J. BERMAN, Senior Program Officer, The John A. Hartford Foundation
LORI BISHOP, Vice President of Palliative and Advanced Care, National Hospice and Palliative Care Organization
PATRICIA A. BOMBA, Vice President and Medical Director, Geriatrics, Excellus BlueCross BlueShield
SUSAN BROWN, Senior Director, Health Education, Susan G. Komen
GRACE B. CAMPBELL, Assistant Professor, Department of Acute and Tertiary Care, University of Pittsburgh School of Nursing, representing the Association of Rehabilitation Nurses
STEVE CLAUSER, Program Director, Improving Healthcare Systems, Patient-Centered Outcomes Research Institute
JEFF COHN, Medical Director, Common Practice
PATRICK CONWAY, President and Chief Executive Officer, Blue Cross and Blue Shield of North Carolina
DAVID J. DEBONO, National Medical Director for Oncology, Anthem, Inc.

---

[1] The National Academies of Sciences, Engineering, and Medicine's forums and roundtables do not issue, review, or approve individual documents. The responsibility for the published Proceedings of a Workshop rests with the workshop rapporteurs and the institution.

CHRISTOPHER M. DEZII, Lead, Quality and Measure Development, State and Federal Payment Agencies, U.S. Value, Access and Payment, Bristol-Myers Squibb
ANDREW DREYFUS, President and Chief Executive Officer, Blue Cross Blue Shield of Massachusetts
CAROLE REDDING FLAMM, Executive Medical Director, Office of Clinical Affairs, Blue Cross Blue Shield Association
MARK B. GANZ, President and Chief Executive Officer, Cambia Health Solutions
ZIAD R. HAYDAR, Senior Vice President and Chief Clinical Officer, Ascension Health
PAMELA S. HINDS, Director of Nursing Research and Quality Outcomes, Children's National Health System
HAIDEN HUSKAMP, 30th Anniversary Professor of Health Care Policy, Harvard Medical School
KIMBERLY JOHNSON, Associate Professor of Medicine, Senior Fellow in the Center for the Study of Aging and Human Development, Duke University School of Medicine
CHARLES N. KAHN III, President and Chief Executive Officer, Federation of American Hospitals
REBECCA A. KIRCH, Executive Vice President of Healthcare Quality and Value, National Patient Advocate Foundation
TOM KOUTSOUMPAS, Co-Founder, Coalition to Transform Advanced Care
SHARI M. LING, Deputy Chief Medical Officer, Center for Clinical Standards and Quality, Centers for Medicare & Medicaid Services
BERNARD LO, President and Chief Executive Officer, The Greenwall Foundation
JOANNE LYNN, Director, Center for Elder Care and Advanced Illness, Altarum Institute
DIANE E. MEIER, Director, Center to Advance Palliative Care
AMY MELNICK, Executive Director, National Coalition for Hospice and Palliative Care
JERI L. MILLER, Chief, Office of End-of-Life and Palliative Care Research and Senior Policy Analyst, Division of Extramural Science Programs, National Institute of Nursing Research, National Institutes of Health

R. SEAN MORRISON, Director, National Palliative Care Research Center

BRENDA NEVIDJON, Chief Executive Officer, Oncology Nursing Society

HAROLD L. PAZ, Executive Vice President and Chief Medical Officer, Aetna Inc.

JUDITH R. PERES, Long-Term and Palliative Care Consultant, Clinical Social Worker and Board Member, Social Work Hospice and Palliative Care Network

PHILLIP A. PIZZO, Founding Director, Stanford Distinguished Careers Institute; Former Dean and David and Susan Heckerman Professor of Pediatrics and of Microbiology and Immunology, Stanford School of Medicine

THOMAS M. PRISELAC, President and Chief Executive Officer, Cedars-Sinai Health System

JOANNE REIFSNYDER, Executive Vice President, Clinical Operations and Chief Nursing Officer, Genesis Healthcare, representing the Hospice and Palliative Nurses Association

RACHEL ROILAND, Director, Quality Innovation, National Quality Forum

JUDITH A. SALERNO, President, The New York Academy of Medicine

DIANE SCHWEITZER, Acting Chief Program Officer, Patient Care Program, Gordon and Betty Moore Foundation

KATRINA M. SCOTT, Oncology Chaplain, Massachusetts General Hospital, representing the Association of Professional Chaplains

KATHERINE SHARPE, Senior Vice President, Patient and Caregiver Support, American Cancer Society

JOSEPH W. SHEGA, Regional Medical Director, VITAS Hospice Care, representing the American Geriatrics Society

CHRISTIAN SINCLAIR, Outpatient Palliative Oncology Lead, Division of Palliative Medicine, University of Kansas Health System, representing the American Academy of Hospice and Palliative Medicine

TANYA STEWART, Senior Medical Director, UnitedHealthcare Retiree Solutions

SUSAN ELIZABETH WANG, Regional Lead for Shared Decision-Making and Advance Care Planning, Southern California Permanente Medical Group, Kaiser Permanente

Roundtable on Quality Care for People with Serious Illness Staff

LAURENE GRAIG, Director, Roundtable on Quality Care for People with Serious Illness
SYLARA MARIE CRUZ, Research Assistant
RAJBIR KAUR, Senior Program Assistant
MICAH WINOGRAD, Financial Associate
SHARYL NASS, Director, Board on Health Care Services, and Director, National Cancer Policy Forum
ANDREW M. POPE, Director, Board on Health Sciences Policy

Reviewers

This Proceedings of a Workshop was reviewed in draft form by individuals chosen for their diverse perspectives and technical expertise. The purpose of this independent review is to provide candid and critical comments that will assist the National Academies of Sciences, Engineering, and Medicine in making each published proceedings as sound as possible and to ensure that it meets the institutional standards for quality, objectivity, evidence, and responsiveness to the charge. The review comments and draft manuscript remain confidential to protect the integrity of the process.

We thank the following individuals for their review of this proceedings:

AMANDA BREWSTER, University of California, Berkeley
LEN NICHOLS, George Mason University
ROBYN STONE, LeadingAge
SARAH SZANTON, Johns Hopkins Bloomberg School of Public Health

Although the reviewers listed above provided many constructive comments and suggestions, they were not asked to endorse the content of the proceedings nor did they see the final draft before its release. The review of this proceedings was overseen by **ELIZABETH BRADLEY,** Vassar College. She was responsible for making certain that an independent examination of this proceedings was carried out in accordance with standards of the

National Academies and that all review comments were carefully considered. Responsibility for the final content rests entirely with the rapporteurs and the National Academies.

Acknowledgments

The National Academies of Sciences, Engineering, and Medicine's Roundtable on Quality Care for People with Serious Illness wishes to express its sincere gratitude to the Planning Committee Co-Chairs Joanne Lynn and Judith Peres for their valuable contributions to the development and organization of this workshop. The roundtable also wishes to thank all the members of the planning committee, who collaborated to ensure a workshop complete with informative presentations and rich discussions. Finally, the roundtable would like to thank the speakers and moderators, who generously shared their expertise and their time with workshop participants.

Support from the many annual sponsors of the Roundtable on Quality Care is critical to the roundtable's work. The sponsors include Aetna Inc., Altarum Institute, American Academy of Hospice and Palliative Medicine, American Cancer Society, American Geriatrics Society, Anthem, Inc., Ascension Health, Association of Professional Chaplains, Association of Rehabilitation Nurses, Blue Cross Blue Shield Association, Blue Cross Blue Shield of Massachusetts, Blue Cross and Blue Shield of North Carolina, Bristol-Myers Squibb, The California State University Institute for Palliative Care, Cambia Health Solutions, Cedars-Sinai Health System, Center to Advance Palliative Care, Centers for Medicare & Medicaid Services, Coalition to Transform Advanced Care, Common Practice, Excellus BlueCross BlueShield, Federation of American Hospitals, The Greenwall Foundation,

The John A. Hartford Foundation, Hospice and Palliative Nurses Association, Kaiser Permanente, Susan G. Komen, Gordon and Betty Moore Foundation, National Coalition for Hospice and Palliative Care, National Hospice and Palliative Care Organization, National Institute of Nursing Research, National Palliative Care Research Center, National Patient Advocate Foundation, National Quality Forum, The New York Academy of Medicine, Oncology Nursing Society, Patient-Centered Outcomes Research Institute, Social Work Hospice and Palliative Care Network, Supportive Care Coalition, UnitedHealth Group, and the National Academy of Medicine.

Contents

ACRONYMS AND ABBREVIATIONS   xix

PROCEEDINGS OF A WORKSHOP   1
INTRODUCTION   1
   Organization of the Workshop and Proceedings, 5
PATIENT AND FAMILY CAREGIVER PERSPECTIVE   6
FRAMING THE ISSUES OF INTEGRATING HEALTH CARE
AND SOCIAL SERVICES FOR PEOPLE WITH SERIOUS
ILLNESS: GAPS, CHALLENGES, AND OPPORTUNITIES   14
   Funding Investments in Social Services, 15
   Building a Strong Social Support Infrastructure, 20
   Discussion, 24
EXPLORING THE KEY ROLE AND UNIQUE NEEDS OF
CAREGIVERS   26
   Caregiving for the Seriously Ill: Overview and Impacts, 27
   The Experience of Caregiving for People with Serious Illness, 31
   Policy Considerations, 33
   Caring Across Generations, 36
   Moving Toward a More Supportive Care Delivery Paradigm, 39
   Discussion, 43

INNOVATIVE PARTNERSHIPS AND COLLABORATIONS FOR
INTEGRATING SERVICES 46
    Program of All-Inclusive Care for the Elderly (PACE), 46
    Building a Bridge to Better Outcomes, 49
    Palliative Care and Social Services for the MostVulnerable, 53
    Community Aging in Place—Advancing Better Living for Elders (CAPABLE), 56
    Discussion, 59
EXPLORING POTENTIAL POLICY CHALLENGES AND
OPPORTUNITIES FOR INTEGRATING HEALTH CARE AND
SOCIAL SERVICES NATIONWIDE 62
    Discussion, 66
    Forging a Way Forward, 68
    Closing Remarks, 69
REFERENCES 69

APPENDIX A: Statement of Task 73
APPENDIX B: Workshop Agenda 75

Boxes and Figures

BOXES

1 Key Definitions, 3
2 Suggestions Made by Individual Workshop Participants for Integrating Health Care and Social Services for People with Serious Illness, 7
3 Paul's Story, 54

FIGURES

1 Caregiver tasks and health effects associated with the longitudinal trajectory of care, 29
2 Percentage of older adults with unmet needs, 30
3 Jobs of the future, 38
4 Framework for caregiver interventions, 41
5 PACE Interdisciplinary Team, 48
6 Safety net palliative care, 55
7 Improvement from baseline to follow up, 58

Acronyms and Abbreviations

ACO	accountable care organization
ADL	activity of daily living
CAPABLE	Community Aging in Place—Advancing Better Living for Elders
CARE	Caregiver Advise, Record, Enable Act
CC	chronic condition
CCTP	Community-based Care Transitions Program
CHRONIC	Creating High-Quality Results and Outcomes Necessary to Improve Chronic Care Act [of 2017]
CMS	Centers for Medicare & Medicaid Services
DEM	dementia
EHR	electronic health record
EOL	end of life
FMLA	Family and Medical Leave Act
GDP	gross domestic product

HCBS	home- and community-based services
HCFA	Health Care Financing Administration
HHS	Health and Human Services
HMO	health maintenance organization
IADL	instrumental activity of daily living
IOM	Institute of Medicine
LTSS	long-term services and supports
NHATS	National Health and Aging Trends Study
NSOC	National Study of Caregiving
OECD	Organisation for Economic Co-operation and Development
PACE	Program of All-Inclusive Care for the Elderly
PTSD	posttraumatic stress disorder
RAISE	Recognize, Assist, Include, Support, and Engage Family Caregivers Act
UCLA	University of California, Los Angeles
VA	Department of Veterans Affairs

Proceedings of a Workshop

INTRODUCTION[1]

A growing body of research indicates that social determinants of health, defined by the World Health Organization as "the conditions in which people are born, grow, work, live, and age, and the wider set of forces and systems shaping the conditions of daily life,"[2] have a significant impact on health care utilization and outcomes.[3] Researchers and policy makers in the United States have spent decades exploring and discussing approaches to integrating health care and social services. While no nation has a truly integrated system, many other industrialized nations invest more heavily in social services than the United States, and are more effective in integrating these services with health care. Such integration is seen both as a way to improve quality of care and health outcomes, as well as to control overall

---

[1] The planning committee's role was limited to planning the workshop, and the Proceedings of a Workshop was prepared by the workshop rapporteurs as a factual summary of what occurred at the workshop. Statements, recommendations, and opinions expressed are those of individual presenters and participants, and are not necessarily endorsed or verified by the National Academies of Sciences, Engineering, and Medicine, and they should not be construed as reflecting any group consensus.

[2] These forces and systems include economic policies and systems, development agendas, social norms, social policies, and political systems. For more information, see http://www.who.int/social_determinants/en (accessed September 21, 2018).

[3] See Box 1 for the definitions of other terms referred to in this Proceedings of a Workshop.

health care costs. Indeed, a number of studies have sought to quantify the health gains associated with a range of social service interventions (Bradley et al., 2016). Integrating health care and social services, such as accessible housing, meals and nutrition services, transportation, and caregiver training, is particularly important for those facing serious illness who typically encounter multiple chronic conditions, pain and other symptoms, functional dependency, frailty, and significant family caregiver needs.[4]

In an effort to better understand and facilitate discussions about the challenges and opportunities related to integrating health care and social services for people with serious illness, the Roundtable on Quality Care for People with Serious Illness of the National Academies of Sciences, Engineering, and Medicine (the National Academies) held a full-day public workshop on July 19, 2018, in Washington, DC. The workshop Integrating Health Care and Social Services for People with Serious Illness featured a broad range of experts and stakeholders including researchers, policy analysts, patient and family caregiving advocates, and representatives of federal agencies. To highlight the critical role of family caregivers in caring for people with serious illness, the workshop featured a session devoted to the unique roles and needs of caregivers, who often serve as a bridge between the health care and social services sectors (see Box 1).

The Roundtable on Quality Care for People with Serious Illness serves to convene stakeholders from government, academia, industry, professional associations, nonprofit advocacy groups, and philanthropies. Inspired by and expanding on the work of the Institute of Medicine's (IOM's)[5] *Dying in America* report (IOM, 2015), the roundtable aims to foster ongoing dialogue about crucial policy and research issues to accelerate and sustain progress in care for people of all ages experiencing serious illness.

In his welcoming remarks to the workshop, James Tulsky of the Dana-Farber Cancer Institute and Harvard Medical School referred to several recommendations contained in the *Dying in America* report, including the recommendation that clinicians be reimbursed for having advance care planning discussions with their patients, which was implemented by the

---

[4] For more information, see https://www.commonwealthfund.org/publications/issue-briefs/2018/jan/using-community-partnerships-integrate-health-and-social (accessed October 10, 2018).

[5] As of March 2016, the Health and Medicine division of the National Academies of Sciences, Engineering, and Medicine continues the consensus studies and convening activities previously carried out by the Institute of Medicine (IOM). The IOM name is used to refer to publications issued prior to July 2015.

> **BOX 1**
> **Key Definitions**
>
> **Home- and community-based services (HCBS)** as defined by Medicare, are types of person-centered care delivered in the home and community. HCBS are often designed to enable people to stay in their homes, rather than moving to a facility for care. Programs designed to help those needing care stay at home and in their communities include the Program of All-Inclusive Care for the Elderly (PACE) (CMS, 2016).
>
> **Hospice** care focuses on caring, not curing, and in most cases, care is provided in the patient's home. Hospice care also is provided in freestanding hospice centers, hospitals, nursing homes, and other long-term care facilities. Hospice services are available to patients of any age, religion, race, or illness. Hospice care is covered under Medicare, Medicaid, most private insurance plans, health maintenance organizations (HMOs), and other managed care organizations (NHPCO, 2017).
>
> **Long-term services and supports (LTSS)** refer to care provided in the home, in community-based settings, or in facilities such as nursing homes. LTSS includes care for older adults and people with disabilities because of age; physical, cognitive, developmental or chronic health conditions or other functional limitations that restrict their abilities to care for themselves. LTSS refers to a wide range of services to help people live more independently by assisting with personal and health care needs and activities of daily living such as eating, bathing, getting dressed, taking medication, cooking, and managing money (CMS, 2016).
>
> **New community-based palliative** care models are meeting the needs of those with a serious illness who are neither hospitalized nor hospice-eligible through provision of care in patient homes, physician offices/clinics, cancer centers, dialysis units, assisted and long-term care facilities, and other community settings. Community-based palliative care services are delivered by clinicians in primary care and specialty care practices (such as oncologists), as well as home-based medical practices, private companies, home health agencies, hospices, and health systems (NHPCO, 2018).
>
> *continued*

> **BOX 1 Continued**
>
> **Palliative care** is specialized medical care for people living with serious illness. It focuses on providing relief from the symptoms and stress of serious illness. The goal is to improve quality of life for both the patient and the family. Palliative care is provided by a team of palliative care doctors, nurses, social workers, and others who work together with a patient's other doctors to provide an extra layer of support. It is appropriate at any age and at any stage in a serious illness and can be provided along with curative treatment (NASEM, 2017).
>
> **Serious illness** is a health condition that carries a high risk of mortality AND either negatively impacts a person's daily function or quality of life, OR excessively strains their caregivers (Kelley and Bollens-Lund, 2018).

Centers for Medicare & Medicaid Services (CMS) as of January 2016.[6] Tulsky pointed out that the committee also discussed the siloed U.S. system of social services and health care services. They had recommended that federal, state, and private insurance and health care delivery programs integrate the financing of medical and social services to support the provision of quality care consistent with the values, goals, and informed preferences of people with serious illness (IOM, 2015). Tulsky added that although that particular recommendation has not been implemented, "I think we are prepared to talk about that today. In fact, as we will learn more about today, this is one of the reasons we have such trouble taking care of some of the most important members of our community."

Workshop planning committee co-chair Joanne Lynn, director of Altarum Institute's Center for Elder Care and Advanced Illness, opened the workshop by noting that the idea of integrating health and social services to better meet the needs of those with serious illness is both an important

---

[6] CMS pays for voluntary advance care planning, which helps Medicare patients make important decisions regarding the type of care they receive and when they receive it. For more information, see https://www.cms.gov/Outreach-and-Education/Medicare-Learning-Network-MLN/MLNProducts/Downloads/AdvanceCarePlanning.pdf (accessed October 22, 2018).

and contentious topic. Acknowledging that some important policy changes regarding the integration of health care and social services have been enacted, Lynn argued that much more needs to be done to truly improve care for people facing serious illness.

Organization of the Workshop and Proceedings

The workshop opened with an interview that highlighted the personal lived experiences of a family facing serious illness, the challenges of full-time caregiving, and the difficulty of securing needed social services. This opening session provided the real-world context of the importance of integrating health care and social services for patients and their families.

Session 1 laid the foundation for the sessions that followed, with a discussion of the rationale for integration of health care and social services for people with serious illness. Speakers discussed differences in spending on health care and social services in the United States compared with other nations and how expenditures on social services affect health outcomes. The importance of creating a strong social services infrastructure was also discussed.

Session 2 explored the integration of health care and social services through the lens of family caregivers. The session highlighted the critical role that family caregivers play in providing and arranging for care for those facing serious illness, the unique challenges they face, and the psychological, emotional, physical, and financial impact of caregiving. Speakers also examined the range of supportive services that caregivers need.

Session 3 shifted the focus to innovative partnerships and collaborations, featuring several operational examples of the integration of health care and social services. Speakers highlighted the Program of All-Inclusive Care for the Elderly (PACE), several partnerships with community-based organizations, Community Aging in Place—Advancing Better Living for Elders (CAPABLE), and palliative care programs for vulnerable populations.

The workshop closed with a discussion of the potential policy challenges and opportunities for integrating services from the perspective of former administrators of CMS, CMS's predecessor, the Health Care Financing Administration, and the Agency for Community Living.

Workshop speakers, panelists, and participants presented a broad range of perspectives and insights. This proceedings describes the presentations given and the discussion that took place throughout the day. Generally, each speaker's presentation is reported in a section attributed to that individual, following the flow of the workshop described above. A summary of suggestions for potential actions from individual workshop participants is found in Box 2. The workshop Statement of Task can be found in Appendix A and the workshop agenda can be found in Appendix B. The workshop speakers' presentations (as PDF and audio files) have been archived online.[7]

PATIENT AND FAMILY CAREGIVER PERSPECTIVE

Judith Peres, long-term care and palliative care consultant, clinical social worker, and board member of the Social Work Hospice and Palliative Care Network, opened the workshop with a discussion with MaryAnn and Frank Spitale about caring for their daughter, Andi. She was born with Smith-Lemli-Opitz Syndrome,[8] a disorder caused by a mutation in a gene involved in the body's production of cholesterol and characterized by slow growth before and after birth, multiple birth defects, and intellectual disability. Frank, a retired pharmacist, also suffers from several serious illnesses, including congestive heart failure, chronic obstructive pulmonary disease, rheumatoid arthritis and osteoarthritis, and diabetes.

In introducing the family, Peres remarked that Andi, who celebrates her 35th birthday this year, represents the type of person with serious illness and disability who is living longer than would have been possible in the past because of the quality care her family has provided her. Peres informed the workshop attendees that MaryAnn, Frank, and Andi recently moved out of their longtime home in Michigan and relocated to the Washington, DC, area to live with their other daughter Nicole, due to Frank's worsening health and the family's financial pressures. "MaryAnn and Frank are sharing their journey with us today to help highlight the fact that the lack of access to coordination of supportive services jeopardizes their health and well-being, as well as making it challenging to keep Andi stimulated and happy," explained Peres.

MaryAnn explained that when they left Michigan to live with Nicole and her husband, she knew there might be a waiting list to obtain supportive services for Andi. When they lived in Michigan, Andi was enrolled

---

[7] For additional information, see http://nationalacademies.org/hmd/Activities/Health-Services/QualityCareforSeriousIllnessRoundtable/2018-JUL-19.aspx (accessed August 13, 2018).

[8] For more information, see https://ghr.nlm.nih.gov/condition/smith-lemli-opitz-syndrome (accessed October 26, 2018).

BOX 2
Suggestions Made by Individual Workshop Participants for Integrating Health Care and Social Services for People with Serious Illness

Supporting Patients with Serious Illness and Their Caregivers and Families

- Ensure that navigators, preferably from social services, are available within health providers' offices to help families find the supportive services they need. (Spitale)
- Include resources in hospitals and doctors' offices to assist new parents of children with chronic illness. (Spitale)
- Create a role within a hospital or health care system to submit waivers and applications, and advocate on behalf of patients with serious or chronic illness and their families. (Spitale)
- Invest in a person-centered, family-centered workforce to complement electronic health records (EHRs). (Stone)
- Encourage social workers to serve as advocates for caregivers. (Oliver, Van Houtven)
- Develop and use standardized caregiver assessments for depression, anxiety, and overall health. (Oliver, Van Houtven)
- Improve availability of resources for caregivers, including bereavement care. (Oliver)
- Ensure case management services are available for individuals with serious illness and their family members, and examine how they are functioning, what their capacity for delivering care is, and what challenges they are experiencing. (Wolff)
- Train across all sectors of care, including both the social and medical, on how to talk to caregivers and support their needs, in much the same way that training was needed to engage in end-of-life discussions. (Gupta, York)
- Operationalize an individual-centered framework that starts with social services, with nearly ubiquitous Area Agencies on Aging serving as the point of entry, and then extends to the health care system. (Stone)
- Consider how to transform care delivery to support person and family-centered care to meet the health and social needs of people with serious illness and their families. (Feinberg)
- Develop strategies for engaging diverse communities in conversations around cognitive and other serious illnesses. (Gupta)

continued

BOX 2 Continued

- Prioritize and address the issue of elder abuse through education and support of caregivers. (Greenlee, Simmons)
- Understand that caregiving is a longitudinal experience that changes over time. When thinking about integrating health and long-term care services or support services for caregivers, it is imperative to think about integration from a longitudinal perspective, as well as a point in time perspective, which is the current approach. (Schulz)
- Understand that not all caregivers need help. (Schulz)
- Allow caregivers to access their patient's health portal and allow caregivers and families to upload caregiver- and family-generated health data. (Wolff)
- Appreciate that the most effective interventions to help families of people with serious illness are comprehensive, multi-component, and tailored to the individual circumstances of caregiving and the serious illness being managed. (Wolff)
- Appreciate that caregiver assessments—having a conversation to understand the specific challenges, needs, strengths, and preferences of caregivers—is foundational to using effective interventions. (Wolff)
- Leverage implementation science and develop pragmatic embedded trials in care delivery to address barriers to dissemination of effective caregiver interventions. (Wolff)
- Develop caregiver interventions to focus on organizational system, societal level interventions, and involve organizational and societal level efforts to bridge health care and social services. (Wolff)
- Think about systematic strategies that would make possible the broader engagement of families. (Wolff)
- Create fields within EHRs for more patient-generated health data, such as caregiver, health care power of attorney, and similar information. (Grant, Wolff)
- Identify, work with, and address each individual patient's own motivations, interests, and goals in order to provide services that are truly beneficial. (Szanton)
- Be aware that serving people with complex health care needs requires first meeting their basic human needs before addressing goals of care or medical interventions. (Kennedy)
- Develop an integrated health and social services platform to enable a common, shared plan of care. (Burch, Greenlee)

Involving Family Caregivers in Team-Based Care

- Include social support professionals—such as home health aides and licensed practical nurses—and family members as potential team members in team-based models of care for individuals with serious illness. (Stone)
- Implement the TRIO guidelines on how to involve family caregivers positively and effectively in care decisions and patient care. (Oliver, Van Houtven)
- Appreciate that patient-centered care cannot happen without family-centered care. (Oliver)
- Simplify the process by which family members can receive their own credentials to access a loved one's EHR. (Grant)
- Identify family caregivers' role in the workforce and the factors that affect their care through annual wellness visits, structured fields in the EHR, and inclusion in clinical assessments of patients. One approach would be to allow family caregivers access to the patient's portal accounts. (Wolff)
- Engage family caregivers so they can offer their perspectives and insights in the care process. (Wolff)
- Clarify and legitimize the role of the family caregiver. Assess and respect their capacities, and offer tailored supports for them. (Wolff)
- Develop the capacity to monitor the experience of family caregivers and the nation's progress toward achieving a more family-centered care delivery system that bridges health care and long-term services and supports. (Wolff)
- Train home care workers on how to handle any language and cultural issues that may arise. (Gupta)

Spreading Innovative Models and Programs

- Disseminate effective programs through national associations using robust communication strategies, finance the establishment of those programs in new locations, and expand the types of patients that the program serves. (Graddy, Simmons)
- Give communities with the appropriate mix of leadership from the local health care, social services, behavioral health, and civic sectors the opportunities to innovate and demonstrate what good comprehensive care at the lowest possible cost would look like. (Lynn)
- Promote new models of partnerships by finding a mutually beneficial situation in the arrangement for both organizations. (Maguire)

continued

BOX 2 Continued

- Develop innovation funds for states to think about the training needs of the home care workforce. (York)
- Consider creative financing approaches such as the use of Social Impact Bonds or Pay for Success financing programs. (Matheis, Simmons)
- Appreciate that bringing a program that integrates health care and social services to scale requires a different skill set than either providing care or initial testing of the program. (Szanton)

Exploring Policy Opportunities

- Consider Medicare for all. (Spitale)
- A collective commitment should be made by the United States for a more humane and caring society to address the artificial separation between medical care and social supportive services. (Feinberg)
- Policy makers need to think beyond hospital, clinic, and health care spending to addressing social needs, which may be a more cost-effective strategy for delivering on the promise of good health outcomes for the U.S. population. (Taylor)
- In considering policy options, focus on the specific social services that produce better health outcomes as well as health care savings. (Taylor)
- Develop and implement incentives for health care organizations and providers to pay more attention to social services and social determinants of health in their health programming. (Taylor)
- Turn the argument of whether to fund social services by funneling dollars through the health care system on its head. Target funding to build a strong social support infrastructure in which the medical care system works. (Stone)
- Appreciate that this is a critical time for those involved in research, policy, advocacy, and practice to attain the needed traction to determine, measure, translate, and validate the value proposition that social determinants affect health and should be included in priorities for future evolution of care models. (Miller)
- Create a universal family social insurance program to which everyone would contribute to help every American afford care. Such a program would also provide an infusion of money into the system to support professionalizing and stabilizing the care workforce. (Gupta)
- Work to define supplemental benefits for the high-need population to help yield significant health changes in a sustainable, economi-

- cally responsible, and culturally and linguistically sensible manner. (Simmons)
- Include caregiver challenges and issues on the political agenda. (Lynn)
- Establish a national strategy that integrates and coordinates a range of benefits and workplace supports for family caregivers—such as paid family leave. (Feinberg)
- Prioritize policies to address the unique challenges and impacts of caregiving for the seriously ill. (Schulz)
- Appreciate that spillover effects from a care system that relies on unpaid and untrained family members and friends can become spillover costs. (Van Houtven)
- Consider policy solutions such as providing increased caregiver training, allowing for paid and unpaid family leave, and stipend programs or caregiver allowances. (Van Houtven)
- Recognize that there are conflicting goals and therefore tradeoffs in policies: from a national perspective, policies that help women remain in the labor force while serving as caregivers are good for the overall economy and boost tax revenues. On the other hand, if women stay home to care for loved ones and do not work, adults with serious illness are kept out of nursing homes and emergency departments, which reduces health care expenditures. (Van Houtven)
- Address the policy and institutional issues necessary to design and support community-level institutions in an integrated system of care. (Vladeck)
- Use precise and accurate language when speaking with policy makers. (Greenlee)
- Ensure that pilot programs have plans and funding to support taking them to scale. (Greenlee)
- Allow Medicare to experiment with more functionally based triggers. For example, create a program where once a person uses post-acute benefits, they immediately receive intensive case management and a care plan. (Greenlee)
- Devise effective approaches to blend all of the current funding streams to support effective integration of health care and social services. (Wilensky)
- Focus on the key issues when considering blending funding streams: who controls the funding, how decisions will be made, and the outcomes and reporting requirements. (Wilensky)
- Support provisions that allow more flexibility for Medicare Advantage plans to provide comprehensive care to beneficiaries. (Wilensky)

in day care and received extra services because she was also enrolled in the state's Medicaid program. The state of Maryland denied their application for Medicaid benefits for Andi, however, which meant that MaryAnn was left providing the 24/7 care for Andi with little extra help. "We looked into day programs and the like, but the price was prohibitive," said MaryAnn. "We did hire some licensed practical nurses to help for a couple of hours here and there, but we are still running out of funds."

Between the extra demands of caring for Andi, the family's diminished savings, Frank's illnesses and hospitalization, and the disruption associated with the addition being built on Nicole's house, MaryAnn fell apart. That is when she met Peres, who she credited with helping her cope with the situation and with providing support in getting help for Andi. Eventually, Medicaid informed MaryAnn that Andi could receive benefits if 75 percent of the Social Security benefit she received was spent on medical bills, so the family saved every receipt for 6 months and submitted the required forms.

Time passed, yet even the family's assigned caseworker was unsure if and when the state would approve their request for Medicaid benefits. Over a period of 18 months, MaryAnn and Frank made repeated phone calls, filled out innumerable applications, and endured five different home assessments of Andi, all to no avail. Then, Frank broke a thoracic vertebra while lifting Andi from her bed to her wheelchair, leaving MaryAnn to take on all the physical demands of caring for their daughter.

Fortunately, Andi's Medicaid benefit was finally approved, and she was granted a waiver from the Maryland Developmental Disabilities Administration, which pays for a day program that should eventually provide in-home respite help. The Spitales' journey to receiving benefits for Andi took a total of 21 months. When Frank developed pneumonia and sepsis, he was able to access a home health care benefit, which MaryAnn had learned about during their efforts to obtain benefits for Andi. "A family should not have to ask," said MaryAnn. "We don't even know what we need. The hospital or someone has to present these things to make it a little easier on families."

Responding to a question from Peres about helpful connections the family had in Michigan, MaryAnn responded that for the most part, because Andi had grown up in Michigan, they were centered in the school system, where the school social worker was very helpful. Even when Andi turned 18 and the family had to apply for legal guardianship, the school social worker went to court to support the family. In Maryland, she and Frank had to hire a lawyer and spend $3,000 to file and gain approval for their guardianship application.

In addition to the legal fees, MaryAnn shared that the Spitales spend nearly one-quarter of their income on medical expenses. Frank noted that while Kaiser Permanente, their current Medicare provider, has their electronic health records (EHRs) available system-wide, Andi's medical records were not shared among the different departments within the Maryland Health Department, which resulted in her having to undergo multiple assessments before receiving her Medicaid benefit. MaryAnn remarked that the process is so intrusive that she believes many people give up in frustration.

Peres asked MaryAnn if she was able to get out of the house during the long period waiting for her daughter's benefits to be approved. MaryAnn replied that even when she did have some free time, all she wanted to do was take a nap. She stopped exercising, which left her even less able to cope with the stress of caring for both Andi and Frank. Increasingly, she had to rely on her daughter Nicole and her husband for help, which increased the stress level of the entire household.

MaryAnn, Frank, and Andi now live in an in-law suite that Nicole and her husband added on to their house after the family moved from Michigan. The addition includes two bedrooms, a family room, a kitchenette, and a roll-in shower for Andi, with no steps or ramps to negotiate. Frank noted that he and MaryAnn had to spend $900 for a roll-in shower chair. MaryAnn added that the county in which they live offers tax breaks for home improvements to serve individuals with disabilities, but the requirements are so strict that Nicole decided to forgo applying for them. She also said the family can spend the funds Andi receives from the Maryland Developmental Disabilities Administration on a van conversion when their current van wears out, though that will mean forgoing the day program for a while.

In an attempt to find ways to manage the multiple challenges the family was facing, MaryAnn turned to a number of online caregiver groups for ideas from people in similar situations. She asked the groups, "as family caregivers, what do you think our government should do" to support you? She said that the majority of the responses called for Medicare for All. Some of the caregiver group members shared their concerns over health insurance coverage given that they did not work outside of the home because they were caring for their spouses with serious illness, and were not yet old enough to qualify for Medicare. MaryAnn told the workshop audience that two friends, one in Canada and the other in the United Kingdom, who have children with the same condition as Andi, do not have to worry about health care coverage and costs. They added that they would never be able to handle what MaryAnn goes through in terms of taking care of their special needs child and arguing over insurance coverage. MaryAnn explained that her Canadian friend chose to put her daughter in assisted living, and the family does not have to pay directly for that care. "It seems like we are really behind here," said MaryAnn. "We do need Medicare for all."

MaryAnn underscored that having someone from the social services system serve as an effective navigator would certainly have helped during the 21 months of waiting for services. The caseworker assigned to Andi was very ineffective, said MaryAnn, and often the family received incorrect information about which office to go to and who to contact. "Someone who knew what was going on and how the system works, enough to get help, would be really helpful," said MaryAnn.

During the discussion session, a workshop participant suggested that Frank and MaryAnn could contact one of the local senior centers, which has free durable medical equipment available and might be able to offer other help. Seconding that suggestion, Christian Sinclair of the University of Kansas asked the Spitales how many "good suggestions" they received that subsequently turned into dead ends. MaryAnn replied that they did not get many suggestions at all. Even after telling them about the requirement to document that they were spending 75 percent of Andi's Social Security benefit on medical care, their caseworker was unclear about how the program worked. Searching the Maryland Health Department's website was equally futile, even for MaryAnn, who is skilled at online research. She did note that everyone she dealt with was kind, but provided no real assistance, with the notable exception of the emergency medical technicians who took Frank to the hospital when he came down with pneumonia and the hospital staff that cared for him. She reiterated that having someone to coordinate care and navigate the system would have been a huge help. JoAnne Reifsnyder representing the Hospice and Palliative Nurses Association thanked the Spitales for sharing their story and grounding the workshop in what truly matters. She noted, "Our topic is integrating health care and social services, and you have really set us on an interesting path. You really were the care manager, bringing together health care and social services."

FRAMING THE ISSUES OF INTEGRATING HEALTH CARE AND SOCIAL SERVICES FOR PEOPLE WITH SERIOUS ILLNESS: GAPS, CHALLENGES, AND OPPORTUNITIES

Building on the patient–family caregiver perspective, the workshop's first panel session framed the issues related to integrating health care and social services for people with serious illness. Session moderator Lynn Feinberg, senior strategic policy advisor at the AARP Public Policy Institute, speaking to the Spitales, said, "You reminded us that serious illness and disability impacts the person, as well as the family. That is why we must transform care delivery to support person and family-centered care to meet the health and social needs of people with serious illness and their families."

Reiterating the need for better integration of health care and social services, Feinberg emphasized, "it is time for our country to make a collective commitment for a more humane and caring society to address the artificial separation that we have between medical care and functional needs in daily living." Moreover, she noted it is critical "to address the needs of family caregivers, because as we saw, families are really the integrators of health care and social supports." She argued that value-based strategies and the recent enactment of the Creating High-Quality Results and Outcomes Necessary to Improve Chronic (CHRONIC) Care Act[9] and the Recognize, Assist, Include, Support, and Engage (RAISE) Family Caregivers Act[10] will establish a national strategy for family caregivers that lays the foundation for a more integrated and coordinated range of benefits.

Funding Investments in Social Services

Lauren A. Taylor, a doctoral candidate in health policy and management at Harvard Business School and co-author with Elizabeth Bradley of *American Health Care Paradox: Why Spending More Is Getting Us Less* (Bradley and Taylor, 2013), began her presentation by appreciating the important contribution the Spitales made to the workshop. She noted that her goal was to provide an "overview of the data that supports the need for additional attention paid to social determinants of health and social services."

Taylor noted that the United States spends more on health care services as a percentage of gross domestic product (GDP) than any of the other 34 countries in the Organisation for Economic Co-operation and Develop-

---

[9] For more information, see https://www.congress.gov/bill/115th-congress/senate-bill/870 (accessed September 21, 2018).

[10] For more information, see https://www.congress.gov/bill/115th-congress/senate-bill/1028 (accessed September 21, 2018). As of this publication, the RAISE Act has not been taken up by a House committee, despite passing the Senate in Fall 2017.

ment (OECD).[11] Taylor explained that the paradox she and Bradley were trying to unravel in their book was why this higher spending on the part of the United States did not result in better health outcomes, such as life expectancy and maternal mortality, on a population level (Bradley and Taylor, 2013). The innovative analysis in the book, noted Taylor, involved taking a holistic look at spending on health care combined with spending on social services in areas such as employment, housing, nutritional supports, and so on. Although the United States was the highest spender in terms of health care services alone, when accounting for expenditures on both health and social services combined, or the investments a nation makes to try to produce health for the population, explained Taylor, the United States dropped into the mid-range of other OECD nations, given its lower expenditures on social services (Bradley and Taylor, 2013).

One way to look at these different expenditure levels, noted Taylor, is that the United States spends a significant amount providing care for those who are sick, while other nations spend more on social services that might prevent people from getting sick. Taylor emphasized how this was clear in the experience of the Spitales who encountered obstacles in receiving social services but found that calling an ambulance when Frank was sick led to an immediate response. "If you are sick, we are ready to come in and rescue you . . . it is probably going to be expensive, but it is really high-quality care," noted Taylor. She went on to point out that in the United States, "we do not have a robust strategy for the prevention side." She believes social services are "upstream prevention" measures that also aim to support people when they are ill. She explained that further analyses of data on health and social services expenditures reveal the ratio of social to health spending to be significantly associated with better health outcomes. Higher ratios of social spending to health care spending were associated with lower infant mortality, fewer premature deaths, longer life expectancy, fewer low birth weight babies, and a reduction in adult obesity, asthma, lung cancer, acute myocardial infarction, and type 2 diabetes (Bradley et al., 2011, 2016).

To Taylor, these analyses support the importance of policy makers adopting a broader view that involves thinking beyond the hospital, clinic, and health care spending, to focus on addressing social needs. Doing so, she said, could lead to a more prudent and perhaps more cost-effective strategy

---

[11] U.S. expenditures on health care totaled 17.2 percent of GDP in 2017 compared with the OECD average of 9 percent of GDP. For more information, see https://data.oecd.org/healthres/health-spending.htm (accessed October 26, 2018).

for delivering on the promise of good health outcomes for the U.S. population. She noted that looking at the ratio of U.S. social spending to health care spending at the state level, as measured by Medicare and Medicaid outlays, indicates a similar relationship to better health outcomes as that of the international comparisons (Bradley et al., 2016).

The challenge, identified Taylor, is that the United States spends so much on health care in general, and Medicaid in particular, that few resources are left for the states to allocate to upstream and more preventive social services. "Frankly, it is a vicious cycle," said Taylor, explaining that failing to allocate dollars to social services results in a sicker population, which in turn requires more spending on health care, leaving fewer dollars for social services.

Taylor noted that when discussing her research with policy makers, they wanted to know on a more granular level which particular social services to prioritize based on research and data. Taylor and her colleagues conducted a literature review to identify which social services produced better health outcomes and saved health care dollars. In sharing the results of the literature review, Taylor acknowledged that saving health care dollars might not be the appropriate metric by which to judge social service investments because, as she reasoned later, investments in the social service sector create returns to the health care sector, often in the forms of reduced utilization. With that caveat in mind, she explained that the literature review found three categories of services that have the strongest evidence of health impacts:

- Housing, particularly housing for chronically homeless individuals and integrated housing and health care for families who are homeless;
- Nutrition, particularly the Special Supplemental Nutrition Program for Women, Infants, and Children and home-delivered meals for older Americans; and
- Case management with home visitation for low-income individuals and low-income first-time mothers (Taylor et al., 2016).

Taylor explained that delivering meals for older Americans, for example, is particularly effective as it provides multiple benefits, addressing both nutritional needs as well as social isolation. She also pointed to the importance of home visitation due to the information it provides about an individual's environment that affects his or her health. For Taylor, these studies highlight the "wrong pocket problem," which describes a situation in which those making the investment in a particular area are not recouping the benefit of that investment (Taylor et al., 2016). "That investment creates returns to the health care sector, often in the form of reduced utilization," she said. "One of the big open policy questions," she explained, is how to do a better job of balancing investments and savings.

The challenge, Taylor explained, is to track the impact of a particular intervention—an investment in Meals on Wheels, for example—and align those investments with the associated benefits. She said there have been a series of health policies, on the national and state levels, and promoted by philanthropic organizations "to incentivize health care to pay much more attention to social services or social determinants of health programming." These policies are trying to "make sure that there are health care organizations that are holding financial risk, are really trying to work upstream to prevent people from getting ill in the first place or to keep them from getting worse," she added.

Taylor cited some examples of this type of effort. She described how six health care providers in Portland, Oregon, donated a combined $21.5 million to invest in the construction of 400 low-income or affordable housing units (Flaccus, 2016). Taylor also noted the work of CareMore Health Plan, a California-based, for-profit managed care organization, which created a loneliness intervention program for approximately 1,100 members who self-identified as being either lonely or socially isolated. This intervention included a team of three outreach workers to connect regularly by phone with those in the program; waiting areas repositioned as social spaces where seniors can drop in and "just be there;" and senior-focused gyms at most of its care centers (Lilleston, 2018). When Taylor contacted CareMore's chief executive officer, he informed her that this program has reduced health care utilization usage among those 1,100 members by 15 to 20 percent.[12] "To me, that is a mind-boggling number, just a huge amount of savings from a fairly light-touch intervention," Taylor said. She provided a third example, that of a start-up in Boston called Circulation, which aims to provide transportation for patients to non-emergency health care appointments that a health care organization or medical practice would pay for as a means of increasing revenues by reducing patient no-shows.[13] Taylor noted that the company claims a 70 percent cost savings from an average 68 percent reduction in no-shows (Circulation, 2018).

---

[12] Information was unpublished at the time of this publication.
[13] For more information, see https://www.circulation.com (accessed August 29, 2018).

In Taylor's view, the key policy question is what the most effective way is to fund new investments in social services. The most obvious options, she explained, would be either to fund such investments through the traditional health care delivery system or put new funding directly into the social services delivery system. She pointed out that funding social services through the health care delivery system may be more politically pragmatic, given the tendency to shy away from being seen as "advocating for a larger welfare state" if additional funding went through the social service delivery system. In addition, the health care system has a track record of responsiveness to financial incentives. "We think we have a highly responsive health care system, that we have trained it to jump at all sorts of carrots and sticks," said Taylor, noting that the health care system knew little about readmissions 15 years ago, but once incentives were provided to reduce readmissions, health care systems responded and reduced readmissions significantly. "There is a sense that we can just rejigger the incentives and [health care] will be responsive," she said.

Although accepting that this may be the more pragmatic approach, Taylor shared several concerns she has about taking such a health care–centric approach. In doing so, she cautioned that perhaps "we just have to live with these concerns, be attentive to them, and try to manage them as best we can. On the other hand, we should at least remain open to the fact that there are alternatives." The first concern she raised relates to valuation. "If we let health care set the terms of what an investment in home-delivered meals is worth, it will always, in my mind, be a systematic underestimate of the value of that intervention," she explained. While an investment in improved nutrition has the potential to decrease utilization, which can be measured, the question is how to value that a person is not hungry or socially isolated. "That is never going to be captured in the kind of return on investment calculations that a health statistics or a managed care company makes," warned Taylor. "That is not necessarily their fault, but it is important to recognize that when we let health care set the terms of what social service investments are worth, it is an incomplete picture."

The second concern Taylor raised related to the feasibility of moving money into the health care system to pay for social services. "In many cases, we have seen the money never gets out of the health care system," Taylor explained, referring to a phenomenon commonly called "trapped and vaporized." "You give it to health care and all of a sudden they have lost it along the way," she said, citing the example of the experience of community-based organizations in New York during the redesign of the state's Medicaid program (Helgerson, 2015).

The efficiency of moving money for social services through the fragmented health care system also concerns Taylor. "Why endure all those administrative costs, all of those contracting costs, all of those levels of overhead?" she asked. Finally, Taylor shared that this approach raises equity concerns, given that there will always be individuals who would benefit from social services, but for whom a return on investment cannot be demonstrated. "Those may be the people who are not sick enough," said Taylor. "They have not historically used enough health care services to bump into the high-need, high-cost group for which you think you are really going to be able to create savings." Taylor fears that health care organizations would prioritize delivering social services to those populations that would produce the greatest savings and neglect those who would also benefit.

Building a Strong Social Support Infrastructure

For Robyn Stone, senior vice president of research at LeadingAge, the argument of whether to fund social services by funneling dollars through the health care system needs to be turned on its head. "These dollars need to be building a strong social support infrastructure in which the medical care system works," she said. "It is the system of last resort, not the system of first resort." While that is an ideal approach, Stone noted that she is a pragmatist, so she has been working to move resources from Medicare and Medicaid programs into affordable senior housing and support for a better social services infrastructure. "Some of the models we are working with allow people to stay in their apartments, stay out of hospitals, stay out of emergency departments, have good quality of life, less social isolation, and live there for the rest of their lives without having to transfer to a nursing home," she explained. These models are important because, as the Spitales's story illustrates, people do not live in the medical care system. "They live in the real world, and for 365 days a year they are addressing their social needs," said Stone.

Stone argued that it is imperative to think broadly and take a framework approach that starts with investing in the social infrastructure in which the medical care system works in order to support and address the concerns from patient and family caregivers as noted by previous workshop presenters. "How do we invest in that? If we have to steal it from health care, I am totally happy to do that," said Stone. "If we have a decision that we all want to pay more taxes and invest in it that way, if we want to have public–private partnerships around that, I think that is great," she added.

Whatever the source of funds, the social infrastructure has to be built at the local level, Stone said, but that will only happen when there is an awareness that the system is not ideally organized for people with serious illness, most of whom live in the community. Stone recounted how, on a recent trip to New Zealand, she was working with some hospice providers who have incorporated occupational therapy, physical therapy, and socially oriented therapies to care for seriously ill individuals—those with as much as 2 years left to live. "A very different model in New Zealand, even at the end of life," noted Stone.

In considering the implications of a social services–oriented framework for health care payment and delivery reform, Stone said she believes this effort has been misplaced in terms of spending millions of dollars to add case managers and yet another layer to the existing health care system. "Somehow, we have to figure out how we can have—what we call in the aging network world—a true, single point of entry that starts with the social services system, not the medical care system," said Stone. In particular, she stressed, putting the single point of entry in primary care adds another layer of responsibility on already overburdened primary care physicians. "We ought to have a system that can wrap around and build in the medical care system when we need it, even for people with serious illness," Stone contended.

Noting the changes in investments in the nation's social service infrastructure, Stone pointed out that the Department of Housing and Urban Development has eliminated its Section 202 program that helped expand the supply of affordable housing with supportive services for the elderly. There are "attacks on most of our nutrition programs and serious attacks on our transportation investments, certainly at the federal level, but we also see it at the state level," posited Stone. She remarked that the growing emphasis on team-based care as part of health care payment and delivery reform is missing the boat by focusing on medical professionals and ignoring social support professionals as potential team members.

Stone pointed out that most care provided in home-based settings is delivered by aides, and sometimes licensed practical nurses. "These are the eyes and the ears of the system, and they are very rarely included in teams," she said, noting that certified nursing aides notice changes in their patients much earlier than other health care professionals do. "They know the behavioral issues, the emotional issues, the social support issues. Why are we not including them as part of the team?" she asked. There are also the families, who provide most of the support in this country, who are not included on the teams either. Today, families become de facto case managers who have to assemble their own support teams. Stone pointed out that "in a system that is truly team-based, we would be starting with the person and the family, and typically the first other professional who touches that person, who is the aide."

In her organization's program on affordable senior housing, Stone explained that there is a service coordinator and part-time wellness nurse embedded in housing communities for every 100 residents. The nurse helps these older adults deal with the fragmented health care system.[14] In Vermont, this program has been bending the Medicare cost curve by approximately $1,200 per person and reducing nursing home placements with an investment in a service coordinator and part-time wellness nurse (Kandilov et al., 2018).

Stone pointed out that the infrastructure exists today to operationalize a person-centered, community-based framework that starts with social services, with nearly ubiquitous Area Agencies on Aging serving as the point of entry to other services such as health care. The question that needs answering, she stressed, is how to take advantage of the framework that already exists in the community, of which the medical care system is only one part. "If you ask people what they need in the community, they are going to tell you we need the supports to allow us to be as healthy and as functional as possible in our community for as long as possible," said Stone. She noted that while other countries may spend more on social supports and care, most are not much better than the United States at integrating social and health care, but they are doing a much better job at figuring out what will work in a given community.

The implications of a socially oriented framework for the workforce are critical, emphasized Stone. Although there is a great deal of concern in the health care sector about integrated EHRs, the best interoperable EHRs in the world are not going to be helpful if staff do not know what to do with those records or how to deliver good services, she argued. Unfortunately, the nation has not invested in the type of workforce that can use the available information and create this type of framework for a person-centered, family-centered system.

Stone identified many questions that need to be answered if the nation is going to develop a truly integrated and team-based approach to health care that builds onto a social support framework, including

---

[14] For further information, see http://www.leadingage.org/members/hud-announces-awards-supportive-services-demonstration-grants (accessed September 18, 2018).

- What does that mean in terms of how teams are developed?
- What does that mean in terms of how a health care system invests in team-based approaches to health, how existing social service systems invest in team-based approaches to health, and how professional schools are investing in team-based approaches to health when they are not incentivized to do that?
- What kind of clinical placements are there?
- How many teams are there, and how many students go out as a team into a home?

Stone described a program at Virginia Commonwealth University that embeds interdisciplinary teams in senior housing to gain experience working on teams and ultimately use that experience in the real world (Jones, 2018). Tremendous investment in the workforce is required for this framework to be effective, said Stone. Indeed, such investment is critical if the United States wants to avoid a situation similar to Japan, where the workforce is far from sufficient to support the nation's elderly population.

Concluding her remarks, Stone pointed out that the United States has spent decades discussing approaches to integrate social and health services. While it is true that no system in the world has a truly integrated system, many other industrialized countries invest more in social services and social care, and are more effective in integrating these services with health care, as outlined by Taylor in her presentation. "I think the recent focus on value-based payment strategies that support financing and delivery integration are promising, but I think a lot of the investments have been put in the wrong place," said Stone. "You are not going to get community outcomes that are successful by continuing to put the money through the medical care system. It is absolutely impossible."

Stone pointed out that 25 to 30 years ago, there was a social health maintenance organization (HMO) demonstration that aimed to bring social care and medical care under one roof at four sites around the country (Harrington and Newcomer, 1991). These social HMOs did a good job at bundling financing, but they did not integrate services at all, which Stone attributed to the fact that the social and health systems were not working together, nor did they even know how to (Yordi, 1988). "They did not have the infrastructure to bring people together," said Stone. She pointed out that there are examples around the country where health and social services are integrated, but these are stand-alone instances and not the norm. "The only way that we are going to make it normative is if we start to get investments in the social support infrastructure," she said.

The challenge, explained Stone, will be to redesign the current entrenched system and shift funding into investments in social infrastructure. Making this challenge even more difficult at the national level is the fact that dollars allocated to Medicare and Medicaid cannot be moved to other parts of the economy to rebalance the system. Perhaps that can happen at the state and local levels, added Stone.

Discussion

During the discussion following the presentations, a workshop participant asked about funding for community health worker programs. Taylor pointed out that the biggest issues for community health workers are who manages them, what their roles are on the health care team, and what the metrics are for evaluating what a good community health worker does. She also expressed the concern that as community health workers migrate from community-based organizations as their employers to health care organizations, their work will be standardized and protocols will need to be followed in counterproductive ways. "The value of community health workers to me is actually the relationship, the cultural concordance, their kind of understanding of the ins and outs of people's lived experience in the community," said Taylor. "If health care organizations 'poach' these workers away from community-based organizations, pay them twice as much, but give them a checklist of 15 things to do every time they show up to a door, we may be squeezing out of that role some of the things we went out and sought their experience for in the first place," warned Taylor. Stone agreed with Taylor and noted that the Promotora model[15] has been around for a long time. Stone wondered why the focus is on investing in new jobs in the medical care system when there is an existing community-based infrastructure to build on and strengthen.

Ellen Blackwell with CMS noted that CMS recently expanded the availability of home- and community-based services through Medicare Advantage organizations. She wondered how the panelists felt about the

---

[15] Promotora refers to a health worker model wherein community health workers who are members of a target population are trained to provide culturally appropriate services as patient advocates, educators, mentors, outreach workers, translators, etc. For more information, see https://www.latinohealthaccess.org/the-promotora-model (accessed September 15, 2018).

opportunities in the Medicare program, and how that might change the long-term care landscape on a larger scale. Stone pointed out the difficulty of working out the details in terms of how a supplemental benefit would be defined and put into practice, and determining the incentives within plans. She does not support extending Medicare as a mechanism for long-term services and supports because she sees that as encompassing a broader range of issues than simply medical care. Feinberg noted that she found CMS's decision to be a cause for optimism and hoped that CMS keeps the program simple and avoids making the benefit so complex that people cannot access it.

Tulsky asked the panelists for their ideas on making direct payments to patients and families that would allow them to procure the social services they need without creating new government structures or adding layers to the health care system. Taylor responded that was an interesting approach, which might be more politically expedient than scaling up social services spending and putting money into a community-based system that some view as bloated and mismanaged. She added that the evidence from the global health perspective strongly supports the direct cash transfer approach. While the concern was that people would not know how to spend this money, Taylor noted that study results show that has not been the case (UK Aid and UK Department for International Development, 2011). "The evidence has been that people know exactly how to spend that money to their own family's benefit," said Taylor. Stone noted that, to a certain extent, many current waiver programs do this for home- and community-based services today. "We have evidence from the Cash & Counseling demonstrations[16] that, not only was there no jeopardy in quality, but it was at least as good quality as agency directed spending," said Stone (U.S. Congress et al., 2003). "You skip the administrative cost of having any kind of agency manage the money," she added.

Another workshop participant pointed out that some health care systems are cutting back on social workers to trim budgets, even though clinical social workers help connect families and patients with services, and asked the panel how to best inform health system leaders about the value of social workers when the value does not immediately affect the bottom line. Taylor remarked that the question speaks to the issue of how to bring

---

[16] For more information, see https://aspe.hhs.gov/basic-report/cash-and-counseling-demonstration-experiment-consumer-directed-personal-assistance-services (accessed September 21, 2018).

evidence to bear to demonstrate the effectiveness of social workers and other kinds of staff that coordinate care.

Lori Bishop of the National Hospice and Palliative Care Organization said she appreciated that the panelists spoke to the need for a collaboration between social services and health care, rather than expecting health care to provide all of the social services. Bishop pointed out that the hospice model of care is a team-based model that includes partners within the community to help with home modification, providing meals, and transportation. She asked the panelists how the system could learn from that model and apply it more broadly. Stone agreed and noted that other models could be studied as well. To her, the problem is how to make the lessons from these programs the norm. "I think it is implementation and scalability science that is missing in terms of how you actually move that into systems in the real world," said Stone. Another issue, she identified, is that the incentives in health care are not all aligned with that type of model.

EXPLORING THE KEY ROLE AND UNIQUE NEEDS OF CAREGIVERS

The workshop's second panel session shifted the focus to the caregivers of those with serious illness. As introduced by moderator Jeri Miller, senior policy analyst and chief of the Office of End-of-Life and Palliative Care Research at the National Institute of Nursing Research, the workshop session underscored that families, not just individuals, may face challenges with housing instability, financial resources, accessibility, social deprivation, isolation, stress, food security, and many other social support issues. The family caregiver, which the workshop planning committee defined broadly as a spouse, care partner, parent, son, daughter, extended family member, friend, or volunteer, may share in those needs. As a result, said Miller, "any discussions we have about integrating health care and social support services for one who is seriously ill must also be shaped with a cognizance of the needs of the caregiver." Although this is not a new issue, Miller noted that it is clear that this is a time for those involved in research, policy, advocacy, and practice to attain the needed traction to determine, measure, translate, and validate the value proposition that social determinants affect health and should be included in priorities for future evolution of care models.

Caregiving for the Seriously Ill: Overview and Impacts

Richard Schulz, distinguished service professor of psychiatry at the University of Pittsburgh School of Medicine, began his presentation by noting that although his work has focused primarily on caregiving for older adults, many of the conclusions from that work are applicable to other populations of caregivers.

Schulz pointed out that there are approximately 18 million family caregivers of older adults in the United States who provide the equivalent of at least $234 billion in unpaid care (NASEM, 2016). However, Schulz noted, the gap between the need and desire for family care and its availability is growing, and will become more acute in the future. He cited adverse effects for the caregiver in terms of economics, psychiatric and physical morbidity, and quality of life. While family members caring for their loved ones is nothing new, Schulz noted that the duration, intensity, and complexity of caregiving is different now than it was even a decade ago. Family caregivers currently are performing many of the complex health care services that in the past might have been provided by a professional nurse, such as giving injections or intravenous infusions. Moreover, family caregivers are doing this work without adequate training or support to carry out these tasks, or even an assessment of their ability to perform these tasks. "These are large deficiencies in our system that need to be addressed," he emphasized.

The impacts of caregiving are highly variable, and not all are negative, noted Schulz. Caregivers, for example, report that they find satisfaction in making a difference in someone's life, but many also report negative effects such as emotional distress, depression, anxiety, and other psychiatric issues (Schulz and Sherwood, 2008). Schulz explained that the intensity and duration of caregiving and the older adult's level of impairment are consistent predictors of depression and anxiety that caregivers experience. Other risk factors for caregivers experiencing adverse effects include

- low socioeconomic status;
- high levels of perceived suffering of the care recipient;
- living with the care recipient;
- lack of choice in taking on the caregiving role, poor physical health of the caregiver;
- lack of social support; and
- a physical home environment that makes care tasks difficult.

In addition to the emotional risks, caregivers can face significant financial risks. For example, caregivers often forgo income and career opportunities, which reduce future Social Security and other retirement benefits if they have to cut back on work hours or leave the workforce to care for a loved one. In addition, substantial out-of-pocket expenses for needed services can undermine a caregiver's own financial security. Schulz pointed out that women, caregivers who have low incomes to begin with, and those with limited work flexibility are most vulnerable to these risks (NRC, 2010). Caregiving is a longitudinal experience that typically starts with sporadic care, noted Schulz (see Figure 1). Over time, caregiving grows to include providing instrumental activities of daily living (IADLs)[17] and ultimately assisting with activities of daily living (ADLs)[18] and placement in a long-term care facility. He noted that caregiving tasks are cumulative over time and are not a discreet set. Although caregiving can start out with taking a relative to the pharmacy to pick up a prescription and perhaps checking on the relative or monitoring a medical condition, the caregiver gradually takes on more responsibilities as the loved one deteriorates and requires more support. By the time the person needing care reaches the middle or late stages of caregiving, the caregiver's tasks become extremely intensive and demanding. "It is at that stage where you see the many negative health consequences associated with caregiving," explained Schulz.

He explained that the two main databases he uses were generated by the National Health and Aging Trends Study (NHATS)[19] and the National Study of Caregiving (NSOC)[20] conducted by the Johns Hopkins Bloomberg School of Public Health. Drawing on NHATS data, Schulz identified three populations of people with serious illness: care recipients with dementia, those who are at the end of life and are expected to die within 1 year, and those who have three or more chronic illnesses. As Schulz noted, these categories are not mutually exclusive, and many caregivers have

---

[17] Instrumental activities of daily living are not necessary for fundamental functioning, but enable an individual to live independently and include activities such as cleaning and maintaining a home, shopping, driving or taking public transportation, managing money, preparing meals, and taking prescribed medications.

[18] Activities of daily living are activities in which people engage and include everyday personal care activities such as bathing, dressing, grooming, toileting, eating, and walking, for example.

[19] For more information, see https://nhats.org (accessed October 3, 2018).

[20] For more information, see https://www.nhats.org/scripts/participant/NSOCOverview.htm (accessed October 3, 2018).

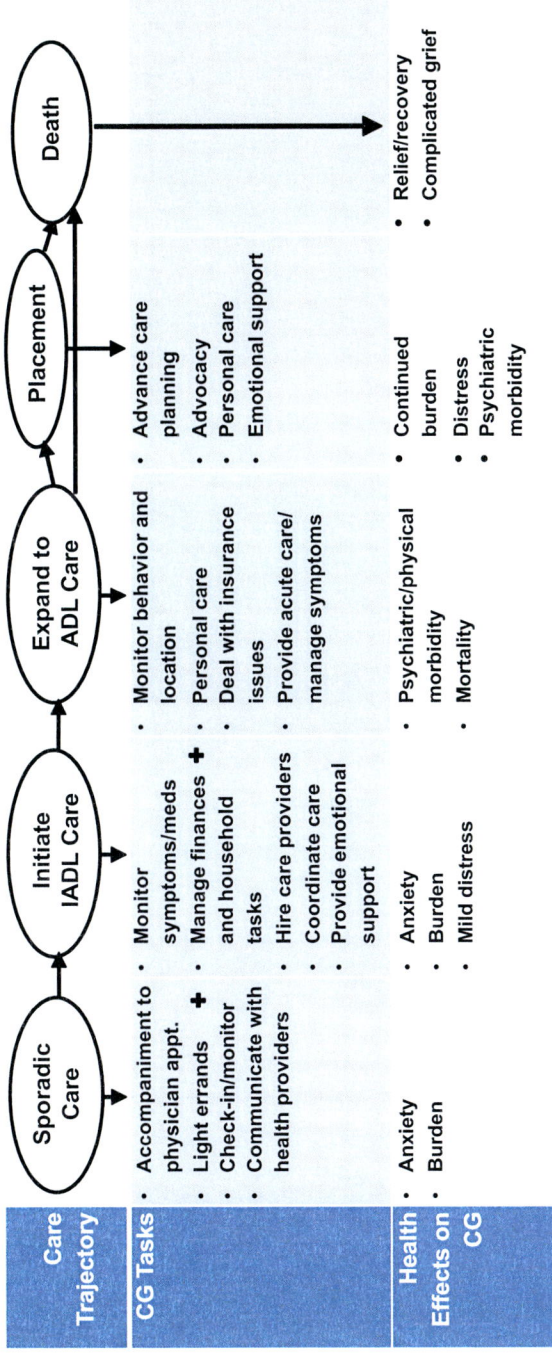

FIGURE 1 Caregiver tasks and health effects associated with the longitudinal trajectory of care.
NOTE: ADL = activity of daily living; CG = caregiver; IADL = instrumental activity of daily living.
SOURCES: As presented by Richard Schulz, July 19, 2018; adapted from NRC, 2010.

to deal with loved ones who have dementia, chronic conditions, and are at the end of life. "That poses challenges even more intense than those that you might imagine occur with individuals caring for persons within one of those categories," said Schulz. According to NHATS data, approximately 290,000 older adults fall in the intersection of those three categories, and 97 percent of those individuals have a family caregiver (Schulz et al., 2018). "As the intensity of the problems increases, the probability of having a caregiver involved also increases," he said.

Schulz described the many ways in which high-need, high-cost patients have a significant impact on the caregiver. As expected, they demand more hours of care, with one-third of caregivers reporting they devote more than 100 hours per month providing care. As the demands for care grow, said Schulz, caregiver psychological and physical morbidity increases, as does the financial strain on the caregiver (Schulz et al., 2018). There are also consequences for the care recipient, particularly regarding the number of unmet needs they experience (Beach and Schulz, 2017) (see Figure 2). For example, individuals with chronic conditions are likely to have wet or soiled clothing; go without bathing, getting dressed, getting out of bed, or going

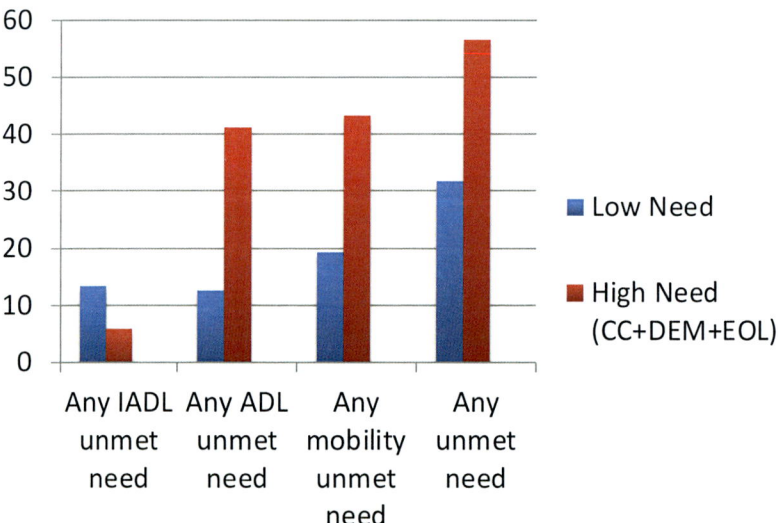

FIGURE 2 Percentage of older adults with unmet needs.
NOTE: ADL = activity of daily living; CC = chronic conditions; DEM = dementia; EOL = end of life; IADL = instrumental activity of daily living.
SOURCES: As presented by Richard Schulz, July 19, 2018; data from Beach and Schulz, 2017.

outside; have limited mobility; and go without hot meals. Those with dementia often have wet or soiled clothes, are bed-bound, and have limited mobility in their homes, while those at the end of life often experience limited mobility in their homes and go without clean laundry (Beach and Schulz, 2017). "The impact of caring for a high-need, high-cost patient not only affects the caregiver adversely, it also feeds back to the patient, resulting in negative impacts in that population as well," said Schulz.

Schulz closed his presentation with three takeaways. First, caregiving is a longitudinal experience that changes over time. As a result, when thinking about integrating health and long-term care services or support services for caregivers, it is imperative to think about it from a longitudinal perspective, as well as a point-in-time perspective, which is the current approach. Second, not all caregivers need help, and many do fine with the challenges they face. Third, caregiving for the seriously ill poses unique challenges and has unique impacts, and addressing those challenges and impacts should be given high priority in terms of policy development.

The Experience of Caregiving for People with Serious Illness

Debra Parker Oliver, the Paul Revare, MD, Family Professor of Family Medicine at the University of Missouri, shared her experience of caring for her husband, David. He was athletic and once rode his bike 72 miles to raise funds to support Alzheimer's disease research. Oliver cared for him as he suffered and ultimately died from nasopharyngeal cancer. Oliver recalled that as she was going through the experience of caring for David, she felt fortunate because she had education, financial resources, and experience in hospice that gave her more resources than most people have. "While this was the hardest thing I ever had to do, it was also the thing that gave me a great deal of pleasure and honor to make sure that the last wishes of the man I loved most in the world were honored," said Oliver.

Highlighting the emotional suffering that comes with the caregiving process, Oliver shared that "you realize in a split second that your world is gone, that nothing is ever going to be the same again, and you do not get to share that with anybody.. . . How could I talk about my guilt, fear, and sorrow in the midst of his dying?" The most intense emotion she experienced was anticipatory grief, which again was something she could not talk about easily with her husband.

Oliver explained that during the 42 months she was her husband's caregiver, there were 18 good months during which the two were able to experience a great deal of joy. "However, it was bittersweet, as you knew that it probably could be your last time," explained Oliver, "and when it was over, I found myself alone for the very first time in my life. Decisions, problems, parenting, and all that sorrow was mine and mine alone." She said she had expected that, because she had experienced so much anticipatory grief that the actual grieving process would be easier. "I guarantee you it is not," she said. She added that if there is a shortage of resources for caregivers the shortage of bereavement care for survivors is more severe.

Oliver shared that in addition to the emotional trauma, the caregiver experiences a number of unwanted transitions. "I liked being David's wife," said Oliver. "I liked him introducing me as the love of his life." Suddenly, she became his primary caregiver, a job she did not ask for, although she was glad to be able to care for him. Speaking about caregivers in general, Oliver said, "Our roles change, our schedules change, our careers are put on hold, and all for an unknown period of time."

Referring back to the Spitales's experience in working to secure benefits for their daughter, Oliver characterized it as a good illustration of the "interactional suffering" families experience when trying to get care for their loved ones. As Oliver explained, interactional suffering results from the lack of attention, understanding, and communication. "Caregivers in our society are invisible," she said. "No one assesses the caregiver. No one asks how you are doing or how you are feeling. No one asks you about your preferences or how much information you want to know. Your questions are not welcome and are often discarded or dismissed." While patient-centered care is a wonderful thing, it cannot happen without family-centered care, and the health care system does a poor job with that, observed Oliver.

The health care system has many gatekeepers to protect busy doctors and nurses, noted Oliver, but that leaves caregivers on their own to figure out when the patient is having an emergency and who to call for help. Making the wrong decision, without training, leads to the patient suffering, she added. Caregivers learn quickly that they must stay on top of things to prevent problems they have to deal with later. "You dare not miss a clinic visit, and you dare not leave during a hospitalization," said Oliver. "Someone is going to drop the ball. Someone is going to do something wrong. Someone is going to withhold or forget a medicine. Some process or some policy is going to stand in the way," she explained.

Oliver commented that a caregiver learns quickly that medicine has limitations but that the language that clinicians use does not reflect those limitations and is not consistent with the way most people use the language.

For example, according to Oliver, "cure," to the average person, means the disease is gone forever, but to an oncologist, "cure" means the cancer is no longer visible on a scan. "I can tell you right now that causes suffering, especially when somebody thinks with their heart and not with their head," said Oliver.

In Oliver's view, some simple steps can make the process easier for caregivers. First, she called for implementation of the Federal TRIO Programs guidelines[21] on how to involve family caregivers positively and effectively in care decisions and patient care and how to manage challenging interactions with family caregivers. These guidelines focus on addressing the policies, practices, and physical environment that lead to interactional suffering (Laidsaar-Powell et al., 2018). "They make caregivers visible and validate their feelings," said Oliver. Second, she called for recognizing that social workers need to be advocates for caregivers, and that having 1 social worker per 80 patients, for example, is insufficient to meet the needs of patients and their caregivers. Third, she noted the importance of developing and using standardized caregiver assessments for depression, anxiety, and overall health. There are tested interventions focused on improving the caregiver experience, Oliver noted.

Concluding her remarks, Oliver hoped the workshop participants would go home with a better understanding of the emotional, physical, and financial challenges caregivers face. Though the health care and social services systems are not to blame for all of these challenges, they do share a responsibility to remedy what they inflict on caregivers. "The fixes are there, and the solutions are not always complex," said Oliver, "and yet nothing is done."

Policy Considerations

Courtney Van Houtven, research scientist in health services research and development in primary care at the Durham, North Carolina, Department of Veterans Affairs (VA), and professor of population health sciences at Duke University, agreed with Oliver's suggestions and the culture change needed to reduce suffering and improve the caregiving experience. She noted that most people do not plan for long-term care, which results in choosing care in an emergency, when quality is difficult to discern.

---

[21] For more information, see https://www2.ed.gov/about/offices/list/ope/trio/index.html (accessed September 21, 2018).

Caregivers, said Van Houtven, are the backbone of the U.S. long-term care system, with nearly 90 percent of older adults with serious illness receiving help exclusively from family and friends. Caregivers operate in isolation, however, and rarely have formal help in the home, even for those patients who are most disabled. Caregivers provide both high- and low-skilled care, yet her research has shown that approximately half of all caregivers have unmet training needs (Van Houtven et al., 2010b). Van Houtven explained that while family caregiving allows people to be cared for in the home, there are "spillover effects" from a system of care that relies on unpaid and untrained family members and friends to provide necessary care.

Van Houtven pointed to research she and her colleagues have conducted that shows that a policy that increases private long-term care insurance coverage reduces reliance on informal care such as unpaid family caregiving. The spillover effect of this reduced reliance on family members for care was found to be an increase in the subsequent generation's work activity. This increased work activity then spills across many different sectors of the economy (Coe et al., 2015). Some of these spillover effects are positive, such as the fact that informal care leads to decreased nursing home entry, home health care needs, and Medicaid inpatient use (Charles and Sevak, 2005; Van Houtven and Norton, 2004). Informal care provided by family and friends decreases Medicare and Medicaid inpatient costs and Medicare long-term care costs associated with reduced use of skilled nursing facilities and home health aides (Coe and Van Houtven, 2009; Coe et al., 2016). Van Houtven noted there is some evidence that having a family caregiver increases patient self-reported health (Coe et al., 2016). What is difficult to quantify, however, is the intangible reward the caregiver gets from doing a job well done and acquiring new skills that benefit their loved one.

One problem, noted Van Houtven, is that spillover benefits can quickly become spillover costs. For example, if the caregiver is in poor health, the reduction in health care use or cost can quickly turn into increases in use and cost, such as from increased emergency room use by Medicare beneficiaries (Ankuda et al., 2017). In addition, the caregivers themselves can experience increased health care use and costs, not to mention the loss of income that Schulz discussed. For caregivers who have to provide intensive care, drug costs rise, presumably to help treat depressive symptoms and the anxiety that often comes with caregiving (Van Houtven et al., 2005). Caregiving can also negatively affect the caregiver's overall health (Coe and Van Houtven, 2009).

In terms of support for working caregivers, Van Houtven pointed out that

> there is a lot of evidence that caregivers quit work at higher rates than noncaregivers, and retire early, thereby threatening their economic security in old age (Jacobs et al., 2014). They also tend to have very high out-of-pocket costs, especially in long-term episodes of caregiving, such as for young injured members of the military and in cancer caregiving, and have increased debt and reductions in their assets.

Even if they can continue working, caregivers often reduce their hours of paid employment, and particularly in the case of female workers, they may experience reduced wages (Van Houtven et al., 2013). "We have done work that found female caregivers have substantial wage reductions, but male caregivers do not have wage penalties," said Van Houtven. "We need to think of caregiving as a female issue, even though we know there are huge contributions of males, as well, but the penalties do accrue to females." In addition, depressed caregivers tend to miss work more, adding to the burden they experience (Wilson et al., 2007).

Turning to potential policy solutions, Van Houtven cited policies such as increased caregiver training, allowing for paid and unpaid family leave, and stipend programs or caregiver allowances, which would benefit caregivers directly (OECD, 2011). For example, better training might enable caregivers to navigate the health system more effectively, reducing stress and anxiety. Family leave programs might help with coping skills and mood because caregivers might have less stress to deal with, and stipend programs might allow families to bring in the extra help they need but can rarely afford, such as respite care, adult day health programs, and home health aides.

To focus on the potential benefits that sound policies can produce, Van Houtven discussed how paid family leave programs can enhance the positive and minimize the negative spillovers of caregiving for people with serious illness. Citing data from her colleague Megan Skira, Van Houtven said that both paid and unpaid family leave programs are effective in terms of increasing a woman's participation in the labor force, though they do not increase the percentage of females who provide intensive care for their loved ones. By contrast, a caregiver allowance or stipend policy is effective in increasing the percentage of females who provide intensive caregiving, but it reduces labor force participation (Skira, 2015). "We need to consider the tradeoffs in some of these policies because so many caregivers do want to remain working or have significant economic consequences if they are unable to work," said Van Houtven. From a national perspective, policies that help women remain in the labor force are good for the overall economy and boost tax revenues. On the other hand, when women stay home to care for their loved ones, adults with serious illness are kept out of nursing homes and emergency departments, which reduces Medicaid expenditures, and by extension, has a positive impact on the U.S. health care budget. "These two goals are in conflict, so I want us to think about this moving forward when we talk about policies and the tradeoffs we need to consider," said Van Houtven.

Van Houtven emphasized that it is also important to consider a specific caregiver policy as it relates to other long-term care policies that indirectly affect caregivers. For example, she and her collaborators have found that a policy that increases private long-term care insurance coverage reduces reliance on informal care, but also has a spillover effect on the next generation by increasing the work activity of the children in the family (Coe et al., 2015). She also noted that a policy that expands formal home care benefits may or may not reduce informal care but may increase caregiver well-being and care recipient outcomes. In closing, Van Houtven summarized that it is important to consider the spillover effects across many different sectors of the economy and other domains that are quantifiable as well as those that are important to caregivers and those receiving care.

Caring Across Generations

Caring Across Generations is a national movement of families, caregivers, people with disabilities, and aging Americans who are working to transform the approach to caregiving in the United States, explained Sarita Gupta, the organization's co-director. The movement's goals, she explained, are two-fold: to build a much needed care infrastructure that includes access to quality, dignified, affordable care options for families and individuals in recognition of the growing caregiving responsibilities that many families face today; and to create 1 million more quality caregiver jobs with adequate training, a living wage, and benefits.

"We are in a moment where care and caregiving needs are absolutely exploding," said Gupta. "Right now, aging adults, with their stagnant income and diminished savings, are no match for the longer lifespans and the rising costs of treating chronic and serious medical conditions and addressing long-term care needs" (CAG, 2017). At the same time that 4 million aging adults are reaching retirement age each year, the first wave of the Millennial generation is having children, boosting the demand for child care in addition to elder care services (CAG, 2017).

Compounding this expansion of care needs at both ends of the age spectrum is the fact that the nation's approach to caregiving came into being during a time when the U.S. economy functioned on the presumption that women would provide unpaid care in the home. Given that is no longer the reality, the burden of care is falling heavily on family members, and in particular, adults. Gupta explained that she and her husband are among those adults, as they care for both a father with Alzheimer's disease and an 8-year-old daughter. "Like my family, about half the workforce expects to be providing care for elders in the next 5 years, and we do not have the systems in place to support that," noted Gupta (CAG, 2017; Goldman, 2017).

The cost of care for seniors and individuals with disabilities is unsupportable relative to most families' financial resources, noted Gupta. She explained that approximately 75 percent of the U.S. workforce earns less than $50,000 per year, yet the average cost of child care today is more than $20,000 per year and a private room in a nursing home costs an average of $80,000 to $100,000 per year (Goldman, 2017). "The numbers just do not add up," said Gupta. She explained that most people rely on a patchwork of approaches to cover the supports and services they need to age at home, including exhausting personal financial resources and relying on family members and friends. Medicaid, which was never intended to be a long-term care program, has become the default way most Americans pay for long-term care, including home- and community-based services (Goldman, 2017).

In addition to affordability issues, the nation does not have the paid workforce it needs to meet the growing demand for care. Gupta explained that the demand for direct care workers is projected to outpace the combined demand for fast food workers, retail sales clerks, teachers, police officers, and firefighters collectively five-fold by 2024 (Bureau of Labor Statistics, 2018) (see Figure 3). The limited number of home care workers are among the most vulnerable workers in the nation, she said, with the majority being women, people of color, and immigrants who make an average of $13,000 per year (PHI, 2015). In fact, approximately 30 percent of home care workers rely on public assistance for food security, and most rely on Medicaid to cover their health care needs (Goldman, 2017). Home care workers, said Gupta, "have been excluded from most labor protections in this country that all other working people take for granted, so with the demand growing for care, we need to take seriously how we are going to grow and strengthen this workforce."

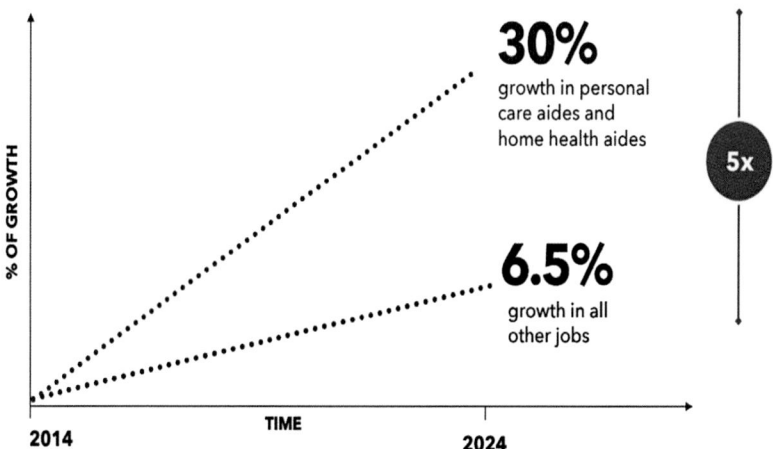

FIGURE 3 Jobs of the future.
SOURCES: As presented by Sarita Gupta, July 19, 2018; graph created by Caring Across Generations with information from the Bureau of Labor Statistics, 2018.

Gupta and her colleagues believe the nation has an opportunity to invest in a better paid, better skilled direct care workforce, which would reduce turnover, improve the quality of life for elders, and reduce costs. To achieve these goals, which would also include the means to help families afford child care and provide paid family care, Caring Across Generations advocates for a universal family care social insurance program to which everyone would contribute and would help every American to afford care. Gupta explained that this program also would provide an infusion of money into the system to support professionalizing and stabilizing the care workforce (CAG, 2017).

While Gupta noted that the ultimate goal is for this to be a national program, she pointed out that some states are already exploring the idea. In November 2018, for example, Maine will vote on the Homecare for All ballot initiative, which would create a dedicated fund to provide in-home care for all seniors, provide supports to family caregivers, and increase care worker wages. She explained that a board composed of caregivers and care recipients would oversee the resulting trust fund, putting what Gupta calls the caring majority—those directly affected by the care system—in charge of decisions about benefits, the workforce, and other aspects of the program.[22]

---

[22] For more information, see https://mainersforhomecare.org (accessed August 29, 2018).

In 2017, Hawaii took a small step toward a universal care program by enacting the Kapuna Caregivers Program, which provides $70 per day to family caregivers who provide care for their aging loved one. Already, Hawaii has doubled the program's budget to $1.2 million in 2018.[23] Washington State's proposed Long-Term Care Trust Act—which would provide a $100-per-day benefit to individuals who need care, in the setting of their choice—gained broad bipartisan support in 2018 and will be proposed again during the 2019 legislative session.[24] Gupta noted that California, Illinois, and Michigan are also studying legislation to support long-term care needs and the associated workforce.

On a final note, Gupta emphasized that the nation clearly needs more affordable and accessible care options for individuals and families. "We have to take seriously the kind of supports that family caregivers need and want, and we have to think seriously about the paid workforce," she said. "We can no longer talk in these spaces and not acknowledge the need for a paid direct care workforce in this country." Ultimately, she added, the key is to develop a broader, more comprehensive approach to the nation's care system, including a universal family care program.

Moving Toward a More Supportive Care Delivery Paradigm

Jennifer Wolff, the Eugene and Mildred Lipitz Professor of Health Policy and Management and director of the Roger C. Lipitz Center for Integrated Health Care at the Johns Hopkins Bloomberg School of Public Health, discussed ways in which the United States can make a difference in the areas of research, policy, and practice to produce a more supportive care delivery paradigm in the future. Wolff first acknowledged that individual clinicians and health care professionals are enormously committed to meeting the needs of individuals with serious illness and their families. "However, the traditional and entrenched care delivery paradigm is not well aligned with the delivery of person-centered care, and is particularly misaligned with the delivery of family-centered care," she noted.

Wolff pointed out, for example, that coverage decisions for reimbursable services are typically predicated on an individual's insurance coverage and do not compensate clinicians and other health professionals for the

---

[23] For more information, see http://www.care4kupuna.com (accessed August 29, 2018).
[24] For more information, see https://www.whca.org/files/2017/12/LTC-Trust-Act-Talking-Acts.pdf (accessed August 29, 2018).

additional time that is necessary to educate, counsel, and support family caregivers. In addition, the prevailing bioethical and legal regulatory frameworks appropriately prioritize individual privacy and the protection of personal health information, yet often lead to challenges for family members who are responsible for coordinating, managing, and overseeing care of individuals with serious illness who lack the capacity to care for themselves.

Moreover, while clinical assessments often ask about the availability of support to bridge functional deficits and cognitive impairment for individuals who require assistance to enact their care plan, these assessments typically do not involve direct interactions with family caregivers. As a result, the information is too often of questionable veracity, and clinicians simply assume that family members will be involved with and capable of caring for their loved one. Wolff added, "a challenge is that because families fall outside formal regulatory, legal, and financial arrangements, they are largely invisible in care delivery." This situation leads to missed opportunities in terms of understanding how to better identify and support families and individuals with serious illness, particularly those who are at risk.

Wolff explained that effective interventions do exist to help families of individuals living with serious illness. The most effective of these interventions, she explained, are comprehensive, multicomponent, and tailored to the individual circumstances of caregiving and the serious illnesses being managed. Caregiver assessment—having a conversation with a purpose to understand the specific challenges, needs, strengths, and preferences of caregivers—is therefore foundational to using interventions that research has shown to be effective. Given the large, robust body of evidence developed through rigorously conducted randomized trials to support these interventions, the challenge is to address the implementation science bottlenecks that lead to few caregivers benefitting from these evidence-based models of care (NASEM, 2016).

One approach to addressing barriers to dissemination of effective interventions, explained Wolff, is to leverage implementation science and develop pragmatic embedded trials in care delivery that focus on engaging at the outset the key stakeholders who would be responsible for diffusing these models. She noted that the National Institutes of Health has been moving forward with this approach in its most recent funding announcements (NIH Collaboratory, 2018).

Referencing the National Academies report *Families Caring for an Aging America* (NASEM, 2016), Wolff called attention to the report's framework for caregiver interventions (see Figure 4). A major takeaway from that

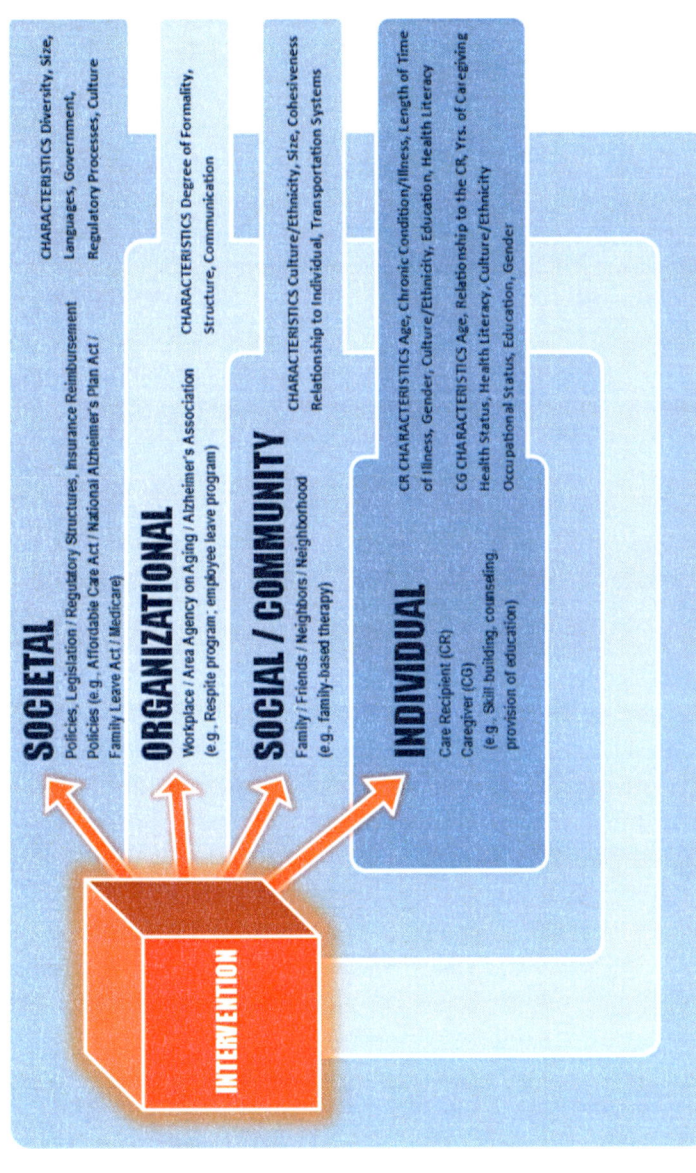

FIGURE 4 Framework for caregiver interventions.
SOURCES: As presented by Jennifer Wolff, July 19, 2018; NASEM, 2016.

report, said Wolff, was that most of the interventions developed to date have focused on individual, interpersonal processes within families, with far fewer focusing on organizational level systems and societal level interventions. Even fewer interventions, she added, involve organizational and societal efforts to bridge health care and social services.

Wolff pointed out that some encouraging payment and delivery reform developments might unfold in the future. "In particular, as we heard earlier with respect to the direct care workforce, there are a number of promising activities at the state level in terms of paid family leave, as well as model legislation that has been developed by AARP around the Caregiver Advise, Record, Enable (CARE) Act to better support family caregivers at the time of hospital discharge," she explained.[25]

Wolff further pointed out that there is a growing awareness at the state and federal levels of the importance of thinking about models that bridge health care and social services. Washington State, for example, is integrating efforts supported by the Administration for Community Living and the National Family Caregiver Support program with its Medicaid programs.[26] In addition, the federal government has taken several promising steps, such as creating new Medicare billing codes that allow clinician reimbursement for non-face-to-face interactions with patients and families that educate and counsel family caregivers.[27] Moreover, Medicaid, said Wolff, is starting to expect that caregiver assessment will occur when the care plan requires involving a family caregiver, and bundled payment models will allow providers the flexibility to innovate and develop new approaches to better support individuals and their family caregivers.

"These developments are, for the most part, providing the opportunity, rather than a mandate, for care delivery to engage families, which we might hope would be moving in the future to thinking about systematic strategies that would make possible engagement of families more broadly," said Wolff. In particular, the RAISE Family Caregivers Act of 2018 sets an expectation that the Secretary of Health and Human Services (HHS) will develop a national plan with multiple private and public stakeholders to

---

[25] For more information, see https://www.aarp.org/politics-society/advocacy/caregiving-advocacy/info-2014/aarp-creates-model-state-bill.html (accessed September 13, 2018).

[26] For more information, see http://www.spokesman.com/stories/2018/mar/05/washington-state-pilot-programs-expanding-support (accessed September 12, 2018).

[27] For more information, see https://www.cms.gov/newsroom/press-releases/cms-proposes-historic-changes-modernize-medicare-and-restore-doctor-patient-relationship (accessed September 12, 2018).

move forward with strategies to better support family caregivers, including monitoring the experience of family caregivers and progress toward achieving that goal.[28]

A national strategy would clearly identify family caregivers so they become a visible part of the workforce and incorporate the family perspective and insights into the care process, explained Wolff. It would also clarify, legitimize, and respect the role of a professional home care workforce, and it would include a deliberative and integrated approach across all care settings and care programs. In addition, a national strategy would include developing the capacity to monitor the experience of family caregivers and the nation's progress toward achieving a more family-centered care delivery system that bridges health care and long-term services and supports (NASEM, 2016).

Discussion

During the discussion session following the panel presentations, workshop participants raised a range of issues. Reverend Amy Ziettlow of the Institute for American Values asked how the Family and Medical Leave Act (FMLA) might help support the seriously ill. Van Houtven replied that although FMLA has a 12-week limit, experience in California has shown that it reduced the number of people with serious illness who used a nursing home. She noted there is some evidence that the Act is helping people remain at home for longer than 12 weeks. "It can really help caregivers perhaps recharge or take care of themselves during that time and not have to juggle work duties and caregiving duties," said Van Houtven. Oliver added that her employer allowed her to take the 12 weeks in pieces rather than all at once, which allowed her the flexibility to use it when she absolutely could not work. However, added Oliver, "if you are an employee at Walmart and you are trying to attend doctor's appointments and be there when a loved one is in the hospital, FMLA is not enough, and those are the people who earn the least amount of money and probably need it most."

Turning the focus to the role of accountable care organizations (ACOs) in improving care for people with serious illness and supporting caregivers, William Blazer of Duke University's Margolis Center for Health Policy commented that one way ACOs may be able to contribute is through their

---

[28] For more information, see https://www.congress.gov/bill/115th-congress/senate-bill/1028 (accessed September 12, 2018).

focus on care coordination and ability to contract with many different partners. He then asked the panelists if they had thoughts on how ACOs can work, either contractually or informally, with community partners to deliver needed services more efficiently. Wolff replied that this is an emerging and important area, one made more complex because families are not currently visible, as noted earlier, in systems of care. In her view, the place to start is with a target population of individuals with serious illness and make a concerted effort to develop data management systems and data capture systems with structured fields that include whether a family member is present and who that family member is. The next step would be to wrap services such as case management around those individuals and family members, and examine how they are functioning, what their capacity for delivering care is, and what challenges they are experiencing. In her view, those steps would move the needle in terms of capturing critical information on who is being served and providing a suitable intervention in a timely manner.

Nguyen Minh Chau from the Montgomery County (Maryland) Commission on Aging and the Vietnamese Senior Association of Long Branch commented on the need to add those suffering from posttraumatic stress disorder (PTSD) to the population of people who may need family support. Van Houtven replied that the VA has a large caregiver support program that serves people with PTSD. "We found a lot of things that we need to do to tailor the caregiver supports for them because they do not like to come into the medical center, as it is very triggering," she explained. "They prefer modes of care that are more online supports through apps, and they also want to have peer support and phone-based supports."

Chau also raised the issue of providing support to help with issues related to language and cultural competency. Schulz said there are a number of interventions that randomized trials have shown to be effective, and many of these interventions have now been translated, adapted for a variety of different populations, and again shown to be effective (Beach et al., 2005; Jongen et al., 2018). In fact, he said, some major interventions developed in the United States for family caregivers are now popular in countries such as China, Germany, and South Korea. "We do have some of the tools and strategies for addressing caregiver needs, and we have evidence showing that they can be reasonably easily translated and applied to populations beyond whites, which is where they typically start out," said Schulz (Belle et al., 2006; Cheung et al., 2015).

Gupta noted that she hears frequently from home care workers about the need for training around cultural competency and managing language issues that arise. In her opinion, given its diversity, the United States needs to develop more strategies for engaging diverse communities in conversations about cognitive and other serious illnesses. She noted that it was a huge challenge getting her community to acknowledge that her father, a retired physician, had Alzheimer's disease.

Amy York with the Elder Care Workforce Alliance commented that training is needed across all sectors of care, including both the social and medical sides of care, on how to talk to caregivers and support their needs, in much the same way that training was needed to engage in end-of-life discussions. Gupta agreed and said incentives are needed to help states figure out how to create such trainings. "I think it would be great if the federal government created innovation funds for states to think about the workforce, the needs, the kinds of training, and the diversity of trainings," she said. "I feel like there is an opportunity right now at the state level to dive into these questions and begin to pilot and model," added Gupta.

Denise Hess from the Supportive Care Coalition asked if the panelists were aware of any best practice examples that use faith community partnerships to address family caregiver needs. Gupta replied that there are a few, though she could not provide details on those projects. Marian Grant from the Coalition to Transform Advanced Care said her organization has worked for years with communities on faith-based efforts for serious illness, both for patients and families. "These are very local experiences and they take a great deal of effort and resources," she said. Many communities, she said, do not have these resources, but the faith community is an appropriate place to look for a partnership, even though it is not always easy for the health system and faith community to work together.

On a different issue, Grant pointed to the difficulty of capturing information about caregivers in the EHR, as well as which individual has health care power of attorney. At the same time, as a clinician, she is not sure what she would do with that information, and she asked the panelists if they had any ideas on how to capture information more effectively on caregivers in the patient record. Oliver said that one reason caregivers are not assessed is precisely because no one knows what do with that information once it is in hand. In most instances, she explained, the caregiver is not a patient of the physician caring for the loved one. Wolff added that her colleagues have been working on improving documentation about caregivers in the EHR, and marking it with visible tabs so it is not lost among the unmarked attachments. She noted that there are advances in the pipeline that would allow more patient-generated health data in the EHR and even allow patients or caregivers to upload information, such as an advance directive they develop with an attorney. Wolff said she is encouraged that most health systems now have the capacity to allow patients to share their electronic health information with their families, which patients often want. What is missing in many cases, she said, is an awareness among the medical community, patients, and families that such access is available. Wolff pointed out that the current registration process for family members to have their own identity credentials is cumbersome and needs to be simplified.

Kathy Greenlee, former assistant secretary for aging at HHS and now at the Center for Practical Bioethics, noted the difficulty of addressing elder abuse, which most often happens at the hands of a caregiver, and the importance of including risk factors for abuse in the assessment of a caregiver. She pointed out that known risk factors for elder abuse include caregiver depression, a care recipient who is combative or resistant to care, and a caregiver who also needs medical treatment. In her view, this issue needs to be prioritized and appropriately addressed through education and support.

INNOVATIVE PARTNERSHIPS AND COLLABORATIONS FOR INTEGRATING SERVICES

In introducing the workshop session on partnerships and collaboration, moderator Peggy Maguire, president of the Cambia Health Foundation, noted that Cambia takes a holistic approach to serious illness care across its foundation, health plans, and strategic technology investments. Among the programs her organization has funded is one that provides counseling and support for caregivers regardless of whether they are insured by Cambia. This program includes an employee resource group for the foundation's employees who are also family caregivers. She noted that this has become one of the company's most popular employee resource groups. Before introducing the first panelist, Maguire said, "personally, I am passionate about helping families prepare for moments of truth and helping people with serious illness live well. It is obvious to me that integrating social and health care services is critical to the equation."

Program of All-Inclusive Care for the Elderly (PACE)

After listening to the previous speakers detail the challenges caregivers face while providing for their family members, Gwendolyn Graddy-Dansby, chief medical officer for PACE Southeast Michigan, pointed out the PACE model addresses many of those challenges. The PACE program works with frail, older adults, a population with the highest medical needs. Graddy-Dansby explained that when she first began working at PACE in 2001, the average age of PACE participants was 85–86. Nearly 20 years later, the average age of a PACE participant is around 73. Regardless of the age of those in the program, Graddy-Dansby emphasized that the PACE model brings together all of the entities the previous speakers had discussed under one umbrella to create a coordinated system of care.[29]

Graddy-Dansby explained that the criteria to quality for PACE include being eligible for nursing home care, being at least 55 years old, and living in the geographic area served by a particular PACE site. At the majority of PACE sites, a large portion of the members is eligible for both Medicaid and Medicare. Once someone enrolls in PACE, the program becomes responsible for all of that individual's care, which means that PACE is capitated for a patient population that is at risk for a number of factors such as hospitalization, drug–drug interactions, disease–drug interactions, and for not receiving care that they need.

Noting that what people want is health, not health care, Graddy-Dansby pointed out that the people who need the most health care—the high-need, high-cost individuals—get the least amount of health. What PACE does to address this conundrum is broaden the model of integrated care by integrating medical care and financing (Eng et al., 1997). "We are the insurer, but also the health care provider, and the benefit of that is it gives us leverage in terms of the types of things we can do, particularly for caregivers," she explained. In addition to integrating medical care and financing, PACE also integrates acute care and long-term care, behavioral health and primary care, and medical and social services. "The interdisciplinary care team," said Graddy-Dansby, "is the sauce that for us works well" (see Figure 5).

The integrated care team, she explained, includes a social worker, a nursing assistant, a home care aide, a nutritionist, and a registered nurse case manager, as well as a transportation coordinator. A physician and nurse practitioner, who are part of the team, play secondary roles to these social components, explained Graddy-Dansby. PACE enrollees have fewer premature nursing home placements and hospitalizations and experience less fragmentation of care, according to Graddy-Dansby. She explained that

---

[29] For more information, see https://www.npaonline.org/pace-you (accessed September 21, 2018).

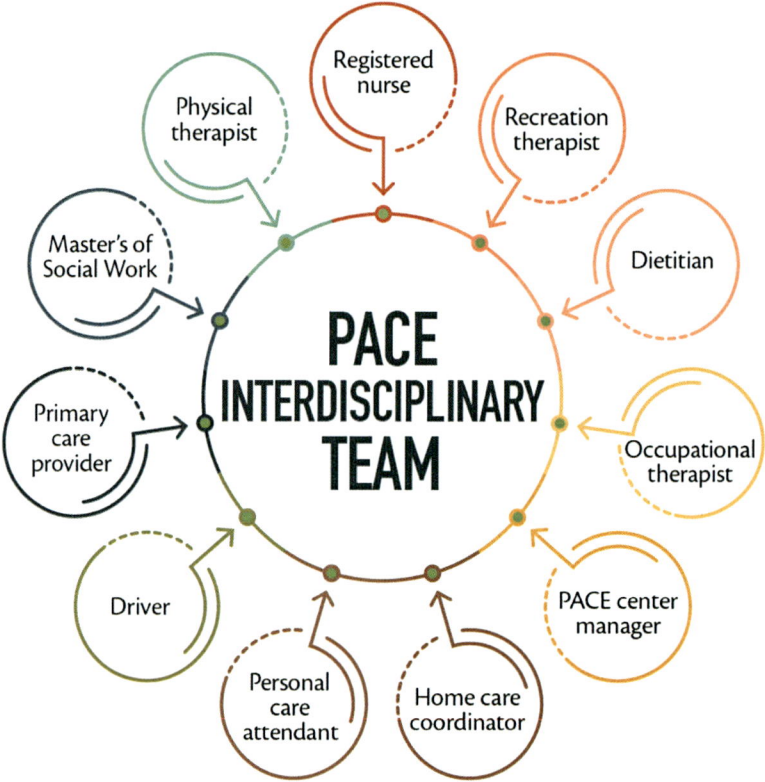

FIGURE 5 PACE Interdisciplinary Team.
SOURCES: As presented by Gwendolyn Graddy-Dansby, July 19, 2018; image credited to the National PACE Association.

PACE may also help to address health disparities. She referenced a study conducted in San Francisco that indicated that older African American adults had better outcomes compared with older white adults enrolled in the program (Tan et al., 2003).

PACE operates on a per member, per month basis rather than a fee-for-service basis, and the program applies its resources to honor what frail elders want, which Graddy-Dansby explained is to stay in familiar surroundings, maintain their autonomy, and maintain a maximum level of physical, social, and cognitive functions. Despite these promising results, PACE has only enrolled approximately 45,000 members out of the roughly 11 million older adults who are eligible for both Medicaid and Medicare, the population that includes the majority of PACE enrollees.

One major impediment is that launching a PACE program involves relatively high start-up costs, explained Graddy-Dansby, and another is finding the workforce that has the right skill set to care for the frail elderly and the desire to do so. Another barrier is that older adults on Medicare lose their Part D benefit if they enroll in PACE. She noted that CMS is starting to look at this, and encouraged workshop participants to advocate in support of changing that requirement.

Integrated service delivery is the core feature of PACE, but unlike in other care models, the physician is not the sole focal point when it comes to providing or coordinating services. "For an individual [who] has a particular need, the discipline that can provide that need becomes the primary driver," said Graddy-Dansby.

Looking to the future, Graddy-Dansby noted that the National PACE Association's strategic plan calls for championing the value of PACE, supporting growth beyond the currently eligible population, and advocating for effective regulatory and payment policies. It also calls for supporting PACE's operation quality through education and data, as well as distinguishing and promoting the PACE brand. She pointed out that educating the medical community about the value of PACE will be particularly important, both to secure the needed workforce and to bring new members into the program.

Building a Bridge to Better Outcomes

Focusing on the social and behavioral determinants of health is not new, as community-based organizations have been doing that for years, explained June Simmons, president and chief executive officer of the Partners in Care Foundation.[30] What is new is the understanding—and its reflection in reimbursement and other incentives within the health care sector—that population health management and value-based care can be achieved only by integrating medical care with home- and community-based services that address the social and behavioral determinants of health.

The approach taken by Simmons's organization is to work with what she refers to as "a wide range of human beings, whether they are Promotores or community health workers, coaches, social workers, or community-based organizations that serve as the ears and eyes in the home" for the health care team, gathering data and information not typically shared in a medical setting or encounter. With proper training, noted

---

[30] For more information, see https://www.picf.org (accessed September 21, 2018).

Simmons, these individuals can conduct comprehensive psychosocial and functional assessments, home safety inspections, and fall-risk evaluations. They can also link medication issues with an evidence-based pharmacist intervention; help individuals to prepare advance directives; provide service coordination and connection to benefits and discounts; pay attention to caregivers and help to provide them with education, training, support, and respite; and connect clients with evidence-based health self-management and fall prevention workshops.

Community-based organizations, said Simmons, serving as a bridge to the home, have worked to improve health and functioning at home for decades, and can parlay the trust and community support they have accumulated over those decades into better care for their clients. They are also connected with all of the available resources in their communities and can help mobilize them without having to reorganize services to meet the requirements of some external model. Community-based organizations have an appreciation for local cultural and linguistic capabilities as well, she added. The challenge her organization is addressing, along with the Administration for Community Living, the National Association of Area Agencies on Aging, The John A. Hartford Foundation, the SCAN Foundation, the Gordon and Betty Moore Foundation, and several others, is to develop consistent screening to target the need for evidence-based approaches for using community-based organizations and to build funding for these services to be included in order to support better health care outcomes.[31]

Simmons explained that Partners in Care and the other collaborating organizations are targeting the populations that need either short-term care management, help with care transitions, or long-term services and supports. Their goal is to reach those who need help, improve self-care and self-management, meet their community support needs, qualify people for available benefits and programs, improve medication adherence, avoid adverse drug effects, and educate and support caregivers. Accomplishing these goals should reduce inappropriate usage, produce a substantial return on investment, increase member satisfaction scores and member retention, and improve provider satisfaction.

As an example of a partnership that meets the goal of reaching high-risk populations, Simmons described the work her organization has done with the University of California, Los Angeles (UCLA), through the

---

[31] For more information, see https://www.aginganddisabilitybusinessinstitute.org/about (accessed October 3, 2018).

CMS-funded Community-based Care Transitions Program (CCTP).[32] CCTP was designed to test models for improving care transitions from the hospital to other settings and reducing readmissions for high-risk Medicare beneficiaries. From 2013 to 2017, Partners and UCLA Health saw 8,300 patients, who were given a choice of interventions. Patients could choose the Coleman Care Transitions Intervention (a home-based health coaching model) or the Rush University Medical Center's Bridge (telephonic social work) plus Partners' own medication safety intervention, HomeMeds,[33] using a UCLA MYMEDS pharmacist to review and make recommendations to improve the medication regimen. The intervention targets medication issues, Simmons explained, as they are so common, and if not properly addressed, typically lead to increased rates of hospital readmission.[34] Simmons noted that a study that will be published soon found that of the high-risk individuals coming out of the hospital, 99 percent had medication-related problems that needed to be reported to their physicians, and would have increased the odds of readmission. This program, said Simmons, produced an average 34 percent reduction in readmission rate versus baseline across 11 hospitals in three Southern California areas.[35]

Based on the success of CCTP, UCLA Health contracted with Partners to implement a second intervention called HomeMeds*Plus*, which includes HomeMeds as well as an in-home psychosocial, fall-risk, and functional assessment with 30 or more days of follow-through to address unmet

---

[32] For more information, see https://innovation.cms.gov/initiatives/CCTP (accessed October 20, 2018).

[33] HomeMeds consists of (a) a comprehensive in-home inventory of all medications present, including over-the-counter medications and supplements; (b) use of a computerized, evidence-based risk screening tool; and (c) pharmacist review and recommendations to patient and prescribers. For more information, see the Agency for Healthcare Research and Quality Health Care Innovations Exchange profile at https://innovations.ahrq.gov/profiles/care-managers-use-software-aided-medication-review-protocol-frail-community-dwelling (accessed October 22, 2018).

[34] The final evaluation of CCTP found that "30-day post-discharge Part A and Part B expenditures were 17.30 percent (p<0.01) lower among participants than for matched comparisons. After accounting for this site's average per eligible discharge rate, this translated into lower net differences in Medicare Part A and Part B expenditures of $10,771,936 (p<0.01) between participants and matched comparisons" (Mathematica Policy Research, 2017).

[35] A recent study pending publication did a propensity-score matched analysis and found significant improvements in 30-, 60-, and 90-day readmissions and emergency department use.

behavioral health and socioeconomic needs.[36] The intervention involves a social worker or health coach working with a pharmacist who addresses medication issues. According to Simmons, this program has developed an automated system to identify who is at risk of readmission, getting them immediately to an on-site coach who assigns them to a set of interventions designed to reduce readmission, and connects them with a home-based program that identifies potential medication issues. According to UCLA, the post-acute HomeMeds*Plus* intervention, which included their MYMEDS pharmacist, decreased the readmission rate for the total population by 3 percent. Compared with high-risk patients who did not get the intervention, UCLA Health found that HomeMeds*Plus* reduced the readmission rate from 30 percent to 10 percent.[37]

Simmons pointed out that these results warrant efforts to spread this type of program. "Now is the time," she said, "to move this agenda forward." She noted positive movement such as the passage of the CHRONIC CARE Act and the availability of Medicare Advantage Special Needs Plans, which, for the first time, are offering "a subset benefit for high-risk people that opens the door to social determinants of health and self-management." She suggested that one approach might be for the National Academies to help lead an effort to define what would be "the next generation that would be eligible for the supplemental benefit." Simmons explained, "we want the right benefit that yields significant health changes" in a sustainable, economically responsible, and culturally and linguistically sensible manner and also accounts for elder abuse risk. "We can see a whole platform of evidence-based, self-management program resources built out across this country that medicine is not taking advantage of and is not yet partnering with," said Simmons.

Simmons credited the Administration for Community Living, The John A. Hartford Foundation, and the SCAN Foundation with bringing groups together across the country to look at how to build integrated regional delivery systems of home- and community-based services for short- and long-term interventions. She underscored the importance of continuing to develop these systems and to encourage the medical community to collaborate with them.

---

[36] Approximately 300 patients per year participate and are among UCLA Health's ACO and Medicare Advantage plan members and primary care patients.

[37] Information was unpublished at the time of this publication.

Palliative Care and Social Services for the Most Vulnerable

For William Kennedy, senior medical director for advanced illness at CareOregon/Housecall Providers, his 20-year journey to provide better care for those in need began when he was a fourth-year medical student in Boston. His experiences in the city and with the people he saw serve as a reminder that there are people who need care and those who want to provide it, and the challenge is to match the two. He noted how Bill Gates, when transitioning from running Microsoft to doing full-time philanthropy, observed, "All of us here . . . at one time or another, have seen human tragedies that broke our hearts, and yet we did nothing, not because we didn't care, but because we didn't know what to do. If we had known how to help, we would have acted. The barrier to change is not too little caring; it is too much complexity" (Gates, 2007).

Kennedy shared the story of a patient he cared for named Paul (see Box 3). He explained that traditional palliative care consists of three pillars: symptom management, care coordination, and setting goals of care. For a patient like Paul, however, those three pillars do not account for the complexities of his life, his isolation, his difficult history, and his ambivalent goals of care, explained Kennedy. The key to working with and helping Paul, said Kennedy, was to determine the ways in which he needed help by developing a lasting therapeutic relationship with him, in spite of the fact that he had not had a life where he developed the support and relationships that would have helped him. "Much of our work is providing clinical longitudinal, highly skilled interventions where these relationships are built, with the understanding that we walk with people for the duration," said Kennedy (see Figure 6).

In many of the patients CareOregon has served over the years, traumatic life experiences are a key part of history that produces the overlap of behavioral health issues, medical complexities, and social determinant problems. Those experiences, in turn, lead to psychological issues, isolation, estrangement from potentially helpful relationships, and other complexities that make it so challenging to work with individuals such as Paul. Overcoming those challenges, said Kennedy, starts with forming a relationship with these individuals. Relationships—especially long-lasting, durable relationships—can be powerful agents of change, an essential ingredient for helping people, and a stabilizing force in these individuals' lives, noted Kennedy.

Serving people who have complex problems requires first meeting their basic human needs before addressing goals of care or medical inter-

> **BOX 3**
> **Paul's Story**
>
> Will Kennedy shared the story of a patient, a 50-year-old man named Paul who was diagnosed with metastatic lung cancer. Kennedy explained that Paul had a history of leaving the hospital against medical advice, and it was never clear why he did so. Paul had led a difficult life that left him physically frail and after his divorce, he lived alone in a single-room occupancy hotel. Paul had agreed to aggressive therapy for his cancer, as he described it in retrospect, without understanding that such care would never cure his cancer. He also experienced complications during treatment that made his life even more difficult—a heart attack and loss of his housing because he could not pay the rent during his prolonged hospital stay. Eventually, the medical team told him there was nothing more they could do for him, but Paul said he would not go into hospice because he said that was giving up. Kennedy noted that "the question becomes, what do we do with people like Paul, how do we serve them, and how do we meet their needs."
>
> Kennedy explained that CareOregon/Housecall Providers' palliative care team worked with Paul to build trust and promised him that they would be with him until the end. Eventually, Paul began to open up to the care team and explained that his abrupt hospital departures against medical advice were a reaction to memories of abuse by an uncle. Whenever a male nurse would come into his hospital room at night, he explained, it would trigger those traumatic memories and drive him to leave the hospital. Disclosing this information led to his further bonding with the care team, and before he died in supportive housing, he told the team that he used to feel like he was falling and now he was not. Kennedy shared that Paul "experienced a peaceful death."

ventions, which Kennedy explained is too often missing from the way the health care system tries to help individuals such as Paul. To illustrate this point, Kennedy recalled a colleague who had just diagnosed a patient with untreatable stage IV cancer. As the colleague was starting to give this person the bad news, he stopped her and said that was the least of his problems. He was worried about where he was going to sleep that night. "There is an acknowledgment that if these things are not met in sequence, we cannot help people in the ways that they need," Kennedy said.

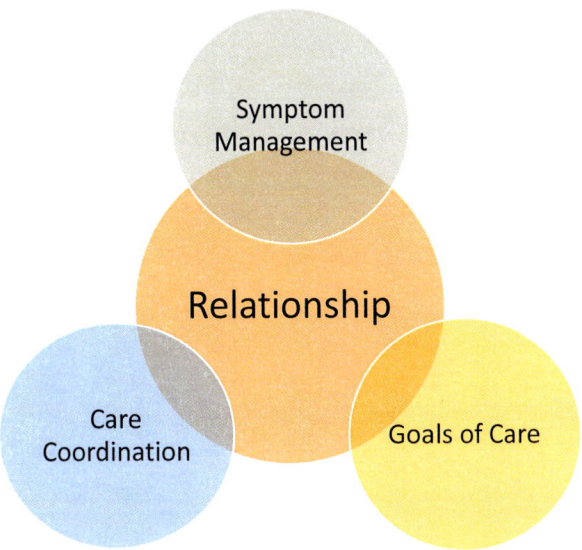

FIGURE 6 Safety net palliative care.
SOURCE: As presented by William Kennedy, July 19, 2018.

Mental health, addiction, lack of social support, food insecurity, housing issues, and health literacy are among the issues that "hit you in the face and jam you when you are trying to take care of these patients," said Kennedy. However, they are only the most visible confounding issues affecting patients such as Paul. There are many other barriers—including lack of insurance, distrust of the system, inaccessible service locations, discrimination, lack of documents or transportation, a disorganized lifestyle, and complex health problems—that keep people from addressing the medical and social services they need. Imagine, he said, being a person in a desperate situation, with multiple complex problems, and not being able to access services because of inadequate identification.

Kennedy cited motivational interviewing as an effective technique for developing a therapeutic relationship with these individuals (Pollak et al., 2011). For people who have lived traumatic lives, he explained, decision making is often a challenge, and motivational interviewing helps to unearth conflicts and bring them to the surface to help people make decisions. Kennedy also uses Advance Care Planning Decisions videos, which are 5- to 7-minute videos that help address the health literacy issue by providing information in plain language and a calm context. "I have seen dramatic differences in applying these tools in our population," he explained.

Kennedy then briefly described a new facility in Portland, Oregon, that CareOregon/Housecall Providers is building. The top two stories of this five-story building will be supportive housing for people who are homeless, and the bottom two floors will be a full-scale, federally qualified health center that will provide primary care, behavioral health care, mental health support, and addiction support. The middle floor will provide supportive housing and medical respite housing for people coming out of the hospital who are homeless. This middle floor will include 10 beds dedicated to end-of-life care for homeless individuals.

Community Aging in Place—
Advancing Better Living for Elders (CAPABLE)

Sarah Szanton, director of the Center for Innovative Caring in Aging at the Johns Hopkins University School of Nursing, began her presentation by noting that when she was a house calls nurse practitioner, she often saw how much a person's home environment affected their ability to care for their chronic conditions. As an example, she told the story of Mrs. B., an elderly African American woman with diabetes, congestive heart failure, high blood pressure, and severe arthritis in her fingers. Mrs. B. spent her days sitting in a chair in a single room in her home. When Szanton and her colleagues first met Mrs. B., the parquet floor of her home had holes in it, making it dangerous for her to move around. She had become so deconditioned that she could not even stand long enough to prepare the food that her grandson brought to fill her refrigerator.

To help individuals such as Mrs. B., Szanton and her collaborators created CAPABLE, a program that features a combination of a nurse, an occupational therapist, and a repair person to address both the person and his or her home at the same time. One unique feature of this program is that it perceives the older adult to be the expert and rather than focusing on his or her chronic conditions, it focuses on what the person wants to be able to do to age at home safely and independently. The team uses its clinical judgment to help the individual devise solutions for addressing pain or depression, as well as any home repair work that might be needed to achieve those goals. This approach, said Szanton, has improved physical function and decreased depressive symptoms in the program's clients. In addition, the program has decreased hospitalizations and nursing home admissions.

The program costs approximately $2,825 per person, with $1,300 budgeted for the repair person (Campaign for Action, 2017).[38]

Szanton described one of the first clients of the program, Mrs. D., who was confused and overmedicated when she was first seen. She spent her entire day sitting in a chair, took 30 minutes to walk to the bathroom, and had not been downstairs in her home for more than 2 years. She could not get out of bed by herself, so her husband would lift her out of bed each morning and place her on a chair that was too narrow for her hips. When Szanton's team was assessing Mrs. D., she said she wanted to be part of the program and that, in addition to getting out of her bed on her own, she wanted to be able to get downstairs and wash her hair in the kitchen sink. "That would not have been any of our goals when we walked in, but that motivated her for strength and independence," said Szanton.

The nurses and occupational therapists who saw her over the next 4 months worked with her to increase her strength and balance in order to reach her goals. In the meantime, the repair person made minor changes to her home, including installing bed risers on the corner of her bed and a firm grab bar for her to use to help her get out of bed. Mrs. D. thought of the idea of placing plastic deck chairs along the hallway so she could practice walking down the hallway by using the chairs as distance markers and a place to rest, as needed. Eventually, she could walk the entire hallway, though she still has a chair at the top of the staircase so she can rest before heading down the stairs. Once she was able to get downstairs, she was also able to be more involved in her family's life. One month after finishing the CAPABLE program, Mrs. D.'s granddaughter called to say the entire family was going to Atlantic City.

In terms of broader results of the program, an assessment of 281 Medicare- and Medicaid-eligible adults ages 65 and older enrolled in CAPABLE found that limitations in ADL improved in 75 percent of these individuals, IADL improved in 65 percent, and depressive symptoms decreased in 53 percent (see Figure 7). Home hazards fell by 77 percent (Szanton et al., 2016). In addition, an evaluation by CMS found that Medicare saved $2,700 per quarter per patient for 2 years after the one-time expense of $2,800 for participating in CAPABLE (Ruiz et al., 2017). Moreover, a study of Medicaid beneficiaries in Maryland found that the program reduced hospitalizations by such a significant amount that it was

---

[38] For more information, see https://nursing.jhu.edu/faculty_research/research/projects/capable/index.html (accessed September 12, 2018).

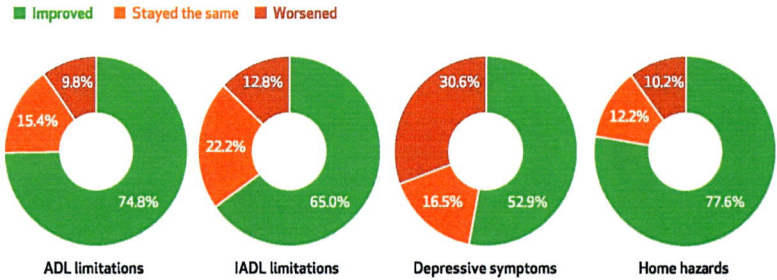

FIGURE 7 Improvement from baseline to follow up.
NOTES: ADL = activity of daily living; IADL = instrumental activity of daily living. The percentages show the shares of participants who improved, stayed the same, or did worse in any category from a baseline level to five-month follow-up. CAPABLE is Community Aging in Place, Advancing Better Living for Elders.
SOURCES: As presented by Sarah Szanton, July 19, 2018; Szanton et al., 2016; authors' analysis. Copyrighted and published by Project HOPE/Health Affairs as "Home-Based Care Program Reduces Disability and Promotes Aging in Place" by Sarah L. Szanton, Bruce Leff, Jennifer L. Wolff, Laken Roberts, and Laura N. Gitlin. *Health Affairs (Milwood)*. September 2016, Vol. 25, No. 9, pages 1558–1563, Exhibit One. The published article is archived and available online at www.healthaffairs.org. Reused with permission from Project HOPE/Health Affairs.

sufficient to pay for CAPABLE services for an entire 1,000-person cohort (Szanton et al., 2018).

Szanton explained that CAPABLE, which started in Baltimore, now operates in 22 states. Blending funding streams has been a challenge, particularly because housing and health care typically are funded through separate streams, but Szanton said the program has been fortunate to identify partners to address that problem. She added that she hopes to be working with the PACE program soon. Szanton pointed out that when she started this program, she believed that if her team could prove that the program saves as much as it costs, everyone would want to participate. "That is not how it works, because it costs money to get started," said Szanton, noting that the level of savings, which is 7 to 10 times the cost of the program, is generating much interest in the program (Ruiz et al., 2017).

Szanton shared some of the lessons learned throughout the course of establishing and operating the program. She said the model is designed to achieve the patient's goals and not the team's goals, and training is needed to get staff in the right mindset to work with CAPABLE clients. "We have mastered how to train people, and we have a combination of online and distance training, but we are going to have to ramp it up to be more accessible throughout the year" as more people become involved in the program, said Szanton. She also learned that scaling requires a different skill set than testing the program. Another lesson was that although health care providers often say they already ask people what they care about, she has learned this is not always the case and that she needs to listen carefully to make sure to ask the appropriate questions to understand fully where an existing program falls short.

Discussion

Maguire opened the discussion by asking Szanton how the CAPABLE model's expansion has been funded. Szanton responded that funding has come from a variety of sources. The Weinberg Foundation has provided funds for expanding the program, and in Michigan, for example, the state's Medicaid waiver program is funding the program. In Boston, the VA is piloting the program, and Szanton hopes to be working with PACE in Massachusetts soon. Several Medicare ACOs around the country are also testing CAPABLE. "It has been a nice mix, and we have been enjoying watching that to see how it works for different kinds of payers," said Szanton.

Graddy-Dansby asked Kennedy how CareOregon/Housecall paid for its new building in Portland. Kennedy replied that all of the health systems in the Portland area contributed funds, as did a large Medicaid and special needs Medicare plan. Central City Concern, the city's largest housing and health care organization serving the homeless, also contributed by using various tax credits and other approaches to raise additional funds. Maguire said that additional funding needs are still being identified, but overall it has been a community-wide collaborative effort.

In response to a request from Maguire to discuss the PACE model in greater detail, Graddy-Dansby recounted the story of one PACE member, a 62-year-old woman with incurable stage IV metastatic non-small cell lung cancer who had never been told that treatment would not cure her cancer. After assessing her health, the PACE staff determined that while she was eligible for hospice, they could give her a good death despite the fact that she had a complicated medical history, including bipolar disorder, issues with opioid abuse, and was taking 21 medications. "We talked to her from day one about comfort care and told her we could not treat her cancer, but we could treat her and give her everything she needs to make her comfortable," said Graddy-Dansby. She agreed to join the program and each of the PACE disciplines—social work, nutrition, behavioral health, spiritual services, transportation, and medical—played an important role in providing this woman with a good death. "We were able to provide all of these resources so that this woman could stay in the community" for the rest of her life, she explained. "This shows how you can take an integrated model of care with a very complicated patient and then make some decisions that improved her quality of life."

Kennedy asked how a new PACE program deals with the possibility that one expensive hospitalization could compromise the entire program. Graddy-Dansby responded that her PACE program faced some of those challenges early on and was fortunate to be part of the large Henry Ford health system, which provided backup financing. What often happens, though, is conversations about appropriate care do not occur when someone first joins PACE. "If those conversations occur, some of those high-cost hospitalizations could potentially be avoided," she explained, either by caring for the person at home or through a short stay in a nursing home.

Cheryl Matheis from the Coalition to Transform Advanced Care commented that the panel described some of the amazing things that can be done when people who understand the financing streams of public programs, foundations, and insurers get creative in the ways they combine funds and functions, and actually save money. She asked if any of the panelists had experience with Social Impact Bonds or Pay for Success financing approaches in which investors put funds into a program demonstrated to save money, and then recoup their investment from those savings. Simmons replied that her organization has not used this financing mechanism, but she met recently with a law firm that has taken an interest in seeing how this type of financing could be used to make health-related investments. "I think those kinds of partnerships could be extremely valuable," said Simmons.

Melissa Williams from the National Patient Advocate Foundation asked how the great examples of community-integrated health and social services could be more widely disseminated. Simmons replied that national associations could play a strong role by publicizing these programs to their members. For example, America's Physician Groups, a national association of managed care physicians, decided that social and behavioral determinants of health are important drivers of population health and important to its members, and is developing ways to help these practices learn about successful programs that address the social and behavioral determinants of health.

It is also developing access pathways to connect with the community groups that can collaborate with them in regional delivery systems. "What is critical is to have that kind of voice that steps up and speaks to this full integration," emphasized Simmons. "Having those credible trusted voices for these kinds of still not fully recognized solutions is a very important form of advocacy."

Williams noted that each of these successful programs was based on partnerships between payers and health systems, and she wondered if such partnerships might represent a way to integrate health and social services. Maguire noted that collaborations among different organizations that previously would see themselves as competitors is absolutely part of the picture. "We are moving to a new world, and I think we need to promote new models and not to promote them as adversaries, but finding the win/win in the arrangement for both organizations," said Maguire.

Graddy-Dansby added that the National PACE Association has been leading the effort to sustain and expand PACE programs and is now developing a best practice guide to further those efforts. For her, the starting point is to identify programs that can show metrics of success, and demonstrate that they do make an impact on both quality of life and utilization. The next step is to identify the components that make that program work, and then disseminate the findings. A workshop participant from the National PACE Association noted that the organization is working on a PACE 2.0 initiative to try to grow and disseminate the PACE model on three fronts. The organization is working with current PACE organizations to glean and disseminate best practices, as well as with communities that are interested in starting a new PACE program, helping them determine how to finance and organize a new program. The organization is also focused on new populations that it can serve with its interdisciplinary care model beyond those who are 55 and older who are eligible for nursing home care. Amy Berman from The John A. Hartford Foundation added that her organization, along with West Health and the Commonwealth Fund, are supporting PACE 2.0 with the goal of expanding PACE to reach 200,000 individuals.[39]

As a closing comment, Szanton noted that the CAPABLE model was funded by a CMS innovation grant. Based on the program's success at improving health while decreasing the cost of care, CMS has asked the CAPABLE program office to write a proposal for CAPABLE to become a

---

[39] For more information, see https://www.npaonline.org/member-resources/strategic-initiatives/pace2-0 (accessed September 12, 2018).

Medicare benefit. "That would be the biggest way of scaling the program," said Szanton.

EXPLORING POTENTIAL POLICY CHALLENGES AND OPPORTUNITIES FOR INTEGRATING HEALTH CARE AND SOCIAL SERVICES NATIONWIDE

The final workshop session focused on policy challenges and opportunities for integrating health care and social services nationwide. Session moderator Joanne Lynn noted that the services available today for caring for people with serious illness are inadequate, unplanned, unreliable, and likely to worsen. "Whatever problems we have now are going to be much worse when we double the number of people [with serious illness] in just the next 15 years," said Lynn (Ortman et al., 2014). She pointed out that when Medicare came into existence in 1965, the average age of death was before 70 and the most common causes of death were heart attack, stroke, and infection (Johnson et al., 2014). Lynn reminded the workshop audience that the average American currently experiences 2 years of self-care disability at the end of life, and 40 percent of older Americans will have some form of cognitive failure by the time they turn 80. Lynn pointed out, "We have not made plans for this even though this is entirely predictable." She noted that approximately 50 percent of Americans now have no income other than Social Security when they retire (SSA, 2017). "How are they possibly going to deal with what they need through 20 to 30 years of retirement, and then have a bad illness?" she asked. "We have done so little to prepare for what is coming at us, and we could still do it if we start today. If we wait until 2035, we are sunk."

Lynn also noted that the medical profession is unprepared for an aging adult population. "How many primary care doctors know the least thing about fitting a cane or about how to deal with the change in the distribution of the drug in the body of the 90 year old?" she asked. "The basics of geriatric care are not even being taught in our medical schools or in our training programs." In addition, she said, changes in immigration policy that restrict the influx of health care workers is going to create severe worker shortages. The problem, she said, is that this issue is not well understood by the public or by the nation's elected officials. "We do not know how to talk to [members of Congress] about the issues of caregiving, and we do not know how to get leadership willing to do anything substantial," said Lynn. Given that research has shown that all kinds of interventions can increase quality of care and reduce costs, the problem is not a dearth of possibilities, but a dearth of will, added Lynn.

In introducing the last workshop panel, Lynn emphasized that the issue is "what can we do now and in the near future that would make it possible for people with serious illness and associated disabilities to live a life that is as meaningful and comfortable as possible at a cost that the community can sustain, that the family can sustain, and that the government can sustain?" She then turned to the session panelists and invited them to share their insights and perspectives.

Bruce Vladeck, senior advisor to the Greater New York Hospital Association, started the session by sharing a few observations based on the day's discussions. In reference to the PACE program, he noted that he has been involved with the program for 40 years and takes "particular pride in the fact that the legislation establishing PACE as a permanent Medicare benefit and permanent state plan option was enacted when I was administrator" of the Health Care Financing Administration (HCFA). Noting that he shares the frustration of others about the continued slow growth of PACE, he pointed out that even if the enrollment could be increased by a factor of 10 overnight, the program would still be reaching only a small fraction of those who are dually eligible and in need of that level of comprehensive care on a regular basis.

Vladeck recalled that when he was HCFA administrator, not 1 day went by when someone did not come to him with an idea they were sure would save Medicare money, but the one thing that most effectively saves Medicare money is to reduce payment rates to providers. "Everything else saves Medicare money in the right kinds of circumstances, and ends up costing more money when a lot of third-rate providers get in and do not target the patients they serve as carefully as the programs we have heard about today," said Vladeck.

He also noted that Szanton's description of CAPABLE was nearly identical to a program his wife worked on in 1983 in Greenwich Village in New York City that is no longer in existence. Indeed, many of the programs discussed during the workshop seemed familiar because he has seen similar programs in a variety of communities. Vladeck said that suggests to him that there is "a policy failure to design or support the kind of institutions that are necessary at the community level to ensure that these kinds of services are available to the people who need them, and that they are good programs, sustainable programs, and that they perform the way they should."

Vladeck emphasized that the burden of running these programs has fallen increasingly on two sets of organizations that are particularly ill suited for the job. "The first are hospitals, which are the last places you want running community-based services or integrating with community-based services as a whole, and I say that as somebody who works for hospitals and is a board member of hospitals," said Vladeck. "We have got to get hospitals out of the focal point of this delivery system." The second are managed care plans, which are already being squeezed financially and do not have the resources to innovate and change the way they function. He added that while there are a few Area Agencies on Aging that could be the integrators of health and social services, the average agency does not have sufficient capabilities or resources.

In addition to the institutional issues that need to be addressed to build an integrated system of care, Vladek noted the financing issue. He argued that the legal and political constraints under which most Medicaid programs operate today mean that when budgets are tight, the only available strategy in dealing with long-term care, realistically, is to cut back on the enforcement of quality standards. "That has been a consistent pattern throughout the 50-year history of Medicaid, financing of long-term care services, and that is not an outcome we want," said Vladeck. At the same time, he believes that even if all of the effective programs were instituted widely, the savings would not make up for Medicare's impending fiscal gap. "We are going to need new ways of paying for this," he asserted. In addition, budget decisions over the past two decades have cut public expenditures on the very social services on which these new programs rely. "I do not see in the current immediate political environment where the revenues are going to come from," said Vladeck.

Vladeck's final point concerned the role of family and other informal caregivers. Given U.S. demographics, the ratio of adult children to all people in need of long-term care is going to fall over the next 20 to 25 years, which means the need for paid caregivers will rise significantly. Noting that he did not have "enough time for my speech" on how the nation is going to have to start treating paid caregivers better, Vladeck emphasized that even at their current inadequate level of compensation, the increased demand for caregivers will cost a great deal of money.

Greenlee built on earlier comments regarding budgeting by noting that it is imperative to tackle the structures that fund these programs. She reminded the workshop that there was a companion piece of legislation, the prevention-focused Older Americans Act, which was passed along with Medicare and Medicaid in 1965.[40] At the time, there was no effort to make relative investments in all three, and instead, Medicare and Medicaid became entitlements and the Older Americans Act did not, which ultimately led to the Administration on Aging's budget being sharply curtailed during the Reagan administration. Greenlee concluded that getting discretionary programs funded is difficult, and because of the structural differences in these programs, it is very difficult to share funding among them. This means that if delivering more home meals saves Medicare or Medicaid money, no formal channels exist to transfer those savings to the Agencies on Aging or the meal providers. "It is not physically possible for a budget structure to pour money from an entitlement program into a discretionary program," explained Greenlee.

In terms of policy opportunities, Greenlee suggested being more precise when conversing with policy makers. "We all talk about cost savings, and from a budget perspective that is an imprecise and inaccurate term," said Greenlee. "We are talking about cost avoidance. When I tell [legislators] that I am going to save them money, they want to spend it." What that means is that asking policy makers to invest in a program today to avoid costs down the road is a hard sell for a legislature struggling with the costs of education and Medicaid, for example, she explained. Greenlee added that long-term investments at the state level also are complicated by term limits imposed on many state legislatures.

Greenlee voiced her frustration with the Center for Medicare & Medicaid Innovation, which funds terrific pilot programs, she said, but lacks plans for scaling programs that do well. She believes the field needs to determine who invests in integrated models of care that can take them to scale. "We need funders, we need state funders, we need foundations, we need advocates to sort of get nerdy about budget policy and understand that we have to have pathways," she said.

The final session panelist, Gail Wilensky, senior fellow at Project HOPE, took exception with Vladeck's comment that the only way to reduce spending is through provider payments, noting that in her opinion, "capitation is the only way to know exactly what will be spent at the end of the day, because you have all of the services covered for a person whereas if you are talking about provider rates you still have the challenge of volume intensity." She then turned to the issue of how to blend funding streams, which she

---

[40] See https://www.acl.gov/about-acl/authorizing-statutes/older-americans-act (accessed September 14, 2018).

said is challenging because of jurisdictional control—both in Congress and in the actual people responsible for the various funding streams—but is conceptually feasible. She noted, though, that making the necessary changes "is much more likely to be a matter of changing law not regulation." She emphasized how important it is to be clear about who, if anyone, has the authority to make change happen and what it would require relative to the current status. For Wilensky, the key questions related to blending funding streams are "who gets control of the funding, how do we make those decisions, what kind of outcomes do we want to require, and what kind of reporting requirements" go along with those outcomes.

Wilensky agreed with the cautionary comments made about putting the health care system in charge of funding social services. "Putting them together is very important, but we have to understand most human nature is to understand what you are trained to do, and if what you are trained to do is to provide medical services, you can be pretty comfortable and quite confident that you will get more medical services when you put them together," said Wilensky. In her opinion, figuring out how to blend all of the current funding streams would go a long way to getting the funding needed to support the kind of effective programs discussed at the workshop. Noting how difficult it would be to accomplish this, she added, "I would just as soon see some of the passion thrown that way," instead of just saying programs need to have more money.

Discussion

Lynn opened the discussion with several provocative ideas for the panel to discuss. The first was to consider giving people living with serious illness the option of giving up their entitlement and entering into a blended funding situation—PACE, for example—with the money that would have gone to Medicaid or Medicare. She also called for ways to energize caregivers to put their challenges and issues on the political agenda. "Up to this point, I would characterize what caregivers have demanded as being crumbs from the table," said Lynn. "I think the caregivers should start demanding things like Social Security benefits. When you have provided 40 hours a week of care to your mother, you ought not to be cut out of Social Security."

She also raised the idea of enabling certain communities to try to create what she called the "Toyota revolution for serious illness care," referring to the Lean process improvement method championed by manufacturing companies such as Toyota and used by health care organizations to improve efficiency.[41] Such communities would have an appropriate mix of leadership from the local health care, social services, behavioral health, and civic sectors who would be given the room to innovate and demonstrate what good comprehensive care at the lowest possible cost would look like.

In response to the first of these ideas, Wilensky questioned whether the CMS administrator has the authority to waive the current statutory prohibition that requires a Medicare recipient to forgo his or her Part D coverage if he or she joins PACE. Lynn said doing so would theoretically involve having the beneficiary pay a fee to the PACE program, which would then buy a market-based plan for that individual. This would be a technical workaround to address a statutory issue, according to Lynn. Wilensky and Vladeck were both of the strong opinion that asking people to give up an entitlement to access a care program was a political non-starter.

In terms of trying new approaches, Greenlee noted that she would like to see Medicare experiment with more functionally based triggers. "I do not think Medicare can afford a long-term care benefit, but I would love it if when someone first begins to use their post-acute benefits that they receive intensive case management and a care plan right then" said Greenlee.

During the question and answer session, Hillary Tsumba from the Primary Care Coalition and the Montgomery County (Maryland) Commission on Aging said she was surprised that the words ageism or ableism were not mentioned during the course of the day, and asked whether those issues come into play when it comes to political will. Greenlee said that what would help most is to have older people advocate for themselves as older people in every venue and every state capital. "That will start to break through ageism and ableism," she said. "We talk about what old people need rather than what do *we* need when *we* get old. We have to have the leadership of older people and encourage them to use their voice." Vladeck added his support to that idea, and Wilensky noted that seniors are an incredibly potent political bloc that votes more often than young people do. In fact, she believes that politicians have been paying more attention to the needs of seniors than they have for preschoolers, for pregnant women, and for people during their early formative years.

Workshop participant John Burch, a self-identified angel investor, suggested that patient-centered repositories of information that integrate data from all kinds of providers, rather than the EHRs housed in health care

---

[41] For example, see http://www.ihi.org/resources/Pages/IHIWhitePapers/GoingLeaninHealthCare.aspx (accessed December 8, 2018).

systems, could serve an important role in integrating health and social services. Greenlee agreed that a platform that integrated health and social services would enable a common, shared plan of care to be more easily developed and shared.

Jennifer Brokaw, an emergency physician, asked how Medicare Advantage plans are able to integrate in-home support of services, based on the idea that they would save money on the total cost care, but that this approach cannot be applied elsewhere. Wilensky replied that she is a strong proponent of the new provisions that allow additional flexibility for Medicare Advantage plans in differentiating benefits for people with different medical conditions (Wilensky, 2018).

Forging a Way Forward

In her final remarks, Greenlee raised the issue of interoperability, noting that in her opinion, meaningful use did not go far enough. She stressed the need for a "commonly shared plan of care, whether that is built up from the provider side, which is where meaningful use has gone, or comes from a portable consumer tool; everyone will need to look at the same game plan." This plan of care is required, she asserted, "in order to really integrate and achieve all that we can in terms of costs savings and health improvement."

Vladeck commented that if the contemporary political realities were put up against demographics and the way the system is working today, the nation would be reading headlines in the next 10 years about older people dying at home, in substandard conditions, because they fell between the cracks. "It is happening now, and we are just not seeing newspaper stories about it, and it is going to happen a lot in the future unless we do something that appears outside the scope of what we are politically capable of," said Vladeck.

Wilensky recounted how when she worked at the White House in 1992, representatives of the Carter Foundation argued that there was enough money being spent on a variety of programs in Atlanta, and that the business and philanthropic communities had committed to provide precisely the kind of integrated services for city residents discussed during this workshop. The problem was that they could not access funding that allowed for flexibility in how it was spent and they wondered if the George H. W. Bush administration could provide that kind of jurisdictional authority. "We tried every which way we could think of to come up with strategies," said Wilensky, who noted that this idea was well received by the

Bush administration. Ultimately, they were unable to develop a strategy to enable them to implement this reasonable approach. Wilensky said, "we are now 25 years later. I can't believe we haven't gotten any closer, but we haven't." Going forward, Wilensky said, "somehow, we have to figure out a way to make that happen."

Closing Remarks

In her closing remarks, Peres thanked all of the speakers for a day full of provocative and insightful discussion related to the integration of health care and social services. As at the start of the workshop, she referred to the IOM's *Dying in America* report, and the committee's recommendation that "federal, state, and private insurance and health care delivery programs should integrate the financing of medical and social services to support the provision of quality care" for people with serious illness. Referring to the discussion in the workshop's final panel, she noted that the committee also emphasized that "to the extent that additional legislation is necessary to implement this recommendation, the administration should seek, and Congress should enact such legislation" (IOM, 2015).

REFERENCES

Ankuda, C. K., D. T. Maust, M. U. Kabeto, R. J. McCammon, K. M. Langa, and D. A. Levine. 2017. Association between spousal caregiver well-being and care recipient healthcare expenditures. *Journal of the American Geriatric Society* 65(10):2220–2226. doi: 10.1111/jgs.15039.

Beach, S. R., and R. Schulz. 2017. Family caregiver factors associated with unmet needs for care of older adults. *Journal of the American Geriatrics Society* 65(3):560–566.

Beach, M. C., E. G. Price, T. L. Gary, K. A. Robinson, A. Gozu, A. Palacio, C. Smarth, M. W. Jenckes, C. Feuerstein, E. B. Bass, N. R. Powe, and L. A. Cooper. 2005. Cultural competency: A systematic review of health care provider educational interventions. *Medical Care* 43(4):356–373.

Belle, S. H., L. Burgio, R. Burns, D. Coon, S. J. Czaja, D. Gallagher-Thompson, L. N. Gitlin, J. Klinger, K. M. Koepke, C. C. Lee, J. Martindale-Adams, L. Nichols, R. Schulz, S. Stahl, A. Stevens, L. Winter, and S. Zhang. 2006. Enhancing the quality of life of dementia caregivers from different ethnic or racial groups: A randomized, controlled trial. *Annals of Internal Medicine* 145(10):727–738.

Bradley, E. H., and L. Taylor. 2013. *The American paradox: Why spending more is getting us less*. New York: PublicAffairs.

Bradley, E. H., B. R. Elkins, J. Herrin, and B. Elbel. 2011. Health and social services expenditures: Associations with health outcomes. *BMJ Quality & Safety* 20(10):826–831.

Bradley, E. H., M. Canavan, E. Rogan, K. Talbert-Slagle, C. Ndumele, L. Taylor, and L. A. Curry. 2016. Variation in health outcomes: The role of spending on social services, public health, and health care, 2000–09. *Health Affairs* 35(5):760–768.

Bureau of Labor Statistics. 2018. *Occupational outlook handbook: Home health aides and personal care aides.* https://www.bls.gov/ooh/healthcare/home-health-aides-and-personal-care-aides.htm (accessed September 9, 2018).

CAG (Caring Across Generations). 2017. *Preparing for the elder book: A framework for state solutions.* New York: Caring Across Generations.

Campaign for Action. 2017. The CAPABLE program: Improving patient outcomes for seniors with low incomes. https://campaignforaction.org/capable-program-improving-patient-outcomes-low-income-seniors (accessed September 21, 2018).

Charles, K. K., and P. Sevak. 2005. Can family caregiving substitute for nursing home care? *Journal of Health Economics* 24(6):1174–1190.

Cheung, K. S., B. H. Lau, P. W. Wong, A. Y. Leung, V. W. Lou, G. M. Chan, and R. Schulz. 2015. Multicomponent intervention on enhancing dementia caregiver well-being and reducing behavioral problems among Hong Kong Chinese: A translational study based on REACH II. *International Journal of Geriatric Psychiatry* 30(5):460–469.

Circulation. 2018. *Circulation health | on-demand NEMT for hospitals, health plans.* https://www.circulation.com (accessed August 29, 2018).

CMS (Centers for Medicare & Medicaid Services). 2016. *LTSS Overview.* https://www.cms.gov/Outreach-and-Education/American-Indian-Alaska-Native/AIAN/LTSS-TA-Center/info/ltss-overview.html (accessed December 3, 2018).

Coe, N. B., and C. H. Van Houtven. 2009. Caring for mom and neglecting yourself?: The health effects of caring for an elderly parent. *Health Economics* 18(9):991–1010. doi: 10.1002/hec.1512.

Coe, N. B., G. S. Goda, and C. H. Van Houtven. 2015. *Family spillovers of long-term care insurance.* Cambridge, MA: National Bureau of Economic Research.

Coe, N. B., J. Guo, R. Konetzka, and C. H. Van Houtven. 2016. *What is the marginal benefit of payment-induced family care?* NBER Working Papers. Cambridge, MA: National Bureau of Economic Research.

Eng, C., J. Pedulla, G. P. Eleazer, R. McCann, and N. Fox. 1997. Program of all-inclusive care for the elderly (PACE): An innovative model of integrated geriatric care and financing. *Journal of the American Geriatrics Society* 45(2):223–232.

Flaccus, G. 2016. 6 Portland health providers give $21.5m for homeless housing. *AP News.* https://www.apnews.com/f4c66b4b23f347e6b1e118b1b3fd8d1c (accessed August 29, 2018).

Gates, B. 2007. Remarks of Bill Gates, Harvard commencement 2007. *The Harvard Gazette,* 2007-06-07.

Goldman, E. 2017. *The caregiver crisis: Rising demand, short supply puts elderly at risk.* https://holisticprimarycare.net/topics/topics-h-n/healthy-aging/1919-the-caregiver-crisis-rising-demand-short-supply-puts-elderly-at-risk.html (accessed September 12, 2018).

Harrington, C., and R. J. Newcomer. 1991. Social health maintenance organizations' service use and costs, 1985–89. *Health Care Financing Review* 12(3):37–52.

Helgerson, J. 2015. *A letter from community and labor about the direction and planning of the DSRIP program.* Commission on the Public's Health System website.

IOM (Insitute of Medicine). 2015. *Dying in America: Improving quality and honoring individual preferences near the end of life.* Washington, DC: The National Academies Press.

Jacobs, J. C., A. Laporte, C. H. Van Houtven, and P. C. Coyte, 2014. Caregiving intensity and retirement status in Canada. *Social Science & Medicine* 102:74–82. doi: 10.1016/j.socscimed.2013.11.051.

Johnson, N., L. Hayes, K. Brown, E. Hoo, and K. Ethier. 2014. *Leading causes of morbidity and mortality and associated behavioral risk and protective factors—United States, 2005–2013.* Atlanta, GA: Centers for Disease Control and Prevention.

Jones, C. W. 2018. VCU receives grant to expand community-based care model for seniors, edited by VCU. Richmond, VA: Virginia Commonwealth University.

Jongen, C., J. McCalman, and R. Bainbridge. 2018. Health workforce cultural competency interventions: A systematic scoping review. *BMC Health Services Research* 18:232.

Kandilov, A., V. Keyes, M. van Hasselt, A. Sanders, N. Siegfried, R. Stone, P. Edwards, A. Collins, and J. Brophy. 2018. The impact of the Vermont support and services at home program on healthcare expenditures. *The Housing-Health Connection* 20(2):7–18.

Kelley, A., and E. Bollens-Lund. 2018. Identifying the population with serious illness: The "denominator" challenge. *Journal of Palliative Medicine* 21:S2.

Laidsaar-Powell, R., P. Butow, F. Boyle, and I. Juraskova. 2018. Facilitating collaborative and effective family involvement in the cancer setting: Guidelines for clinicians (trio guidelines-1). *Patient Education and Counseling* 101(6):970–982.

Lilleston, R. 2018. *Caremore's program aims to treat loneliness amongst 50+.* Washington, DC: AARP.

Mathematica Policy Research. 2017. *Final evaluation report: Evaluation of the community-based care transitions program.* Washington, DC: Centers for Medicare & Medicaid Services.

NASEM (National Academies of Sciences, Engineering, and Medicine). 2016. *Families caring for an aging America.* Washington, DC: The National Academies Press. doi: https://doi.org/10.17226/23606.

NASEM. 2017. *Integrating the patient and caregiver voice into serious illness care: Proceedings of a workshop.* Washington, DC: The National Academies Press. doi: https://doi.org/10.17226/24802.

NHPCO (National Hospice and Palliative Care Organization). 2017. Hospice care. https://www.nhpco.org/about/hospice-care (accessed August 22, 2018).

NHPCO. 2018. Clinical practice guidelines for quality palliative care, 4th ed. National Consensus Project for Quality Palliative Care, 2018. Richmond, VA: NHPCO.

NIH (National Institutes of Health) Collaboratory. 2018. Living textbook of pragmatic clinical trials. http://rethinkingclinicaltrials.org (accessed November 2, 2018).

NRC (National Research Council). 2010. *The role of human factors in home health care: Workshop summary.* Washington, DC: The National Academies Press.

OECD (Organisation for Economic Co-operation and Development). 2011. *Help wanted?: Providing and paying for long-term care.* Paris, France: OECD.

Ortman, J., V. Velkoff, and H. Hogan. 2014. *An aging nation: The older population in the United States.* Washington, DC: U.S. Census Bureau.

PHI. 2015. *Paying the price: How poverty wages undermine home care in america.* Bronx, NY: PHI.

Pollak, K. I., J. W. Childers, and R. M. Arnold. 2011. Applying motivational interviewing techniques to palliative care communication. *Journal of Palliative Medicine* 14(5):587–592.

Ruiz, S., L. P. Snyder, C. Rotondo, C. Cross-Barnet, E. M. Colligan, and K. Giuriceo. 2017. Innovative home visit models associated with reductions in costs, hospitalizations, and emergency department use. *Health Affairs* 36(3):425–432.

Schulz, R., and P. R. Sherwood. 2008. Physical and mental health effects of family caregiving. *The American Journal of Nursing* 108(9 Suppl):23–27.

Schulz, R., S. R. Beach, E. M. Friedman, G. R. Martsolf, J. Rodakowski, and A. E. James, 3rd. 2018. Changing structures and processes to support family caregivers of seriously ill patients. *Journal of Palliative Medicine* 21(S2):S36–S42.

Skira, M. 2015. Dynamic wage and employment effects of elder parent care. *International Economic Review* 56:63–93.

SSA (Social Security Administration). 2017. *Fact sheet*. Washington, DC: SSA.

Szanton, S. L., B. Leff, J. L. Wolff, L. Roberts, and L. N. Gitlin. 2016. Home-based care program reduces disability and promotes aging in place. *Health Affairs* 35(9):1558–1563.

Szanton, S. L., Y. N. Alfonso, B. Leff, J. Guralnik, J. L. Wolff, I. Stockwell, L. N. Gitlin, and D. Bishai. 2018. Medicaid cost savings of a preventive home visit program for disabled older adults. *Journal of the American Geriatrics Society* 66(3):614–620.

Tan, E., L. Li-Ying, C. Eng, A. Jha, and K. E. Covinsky. 2003. Differences in mortality of black and white patients enrolled in the program of all-inclusive care for the elderly. *Journal of the American Geriatrics Society* 51:246–251.

Taylor, L. A., A. X. Tan, C. E. Coyle, C. Ndumele, E. Rogan, M. Canavan, L. A. Curry, and E. H. Bradley. 2016. Leveraging the social determinants of health: What works? *PLoS ONE* 11(8):e0160217.

UK Aid and UK Department for International Development. 2011. *DFID cash transfers evidence paper*. Geneva, Switzerland: World Health Organization.

U.S. Congress, House of Representatives. Subcommittee on Health of the Committee on Energy and Commerce. 2003. *Consumer directed services: Improving medicaid beneficiaries' access to quality care*. 1st Session. June 5, 2003.

Van Houtven, C., and E. C. Norton. 2004. Informal care and health care use of older adults. *Journal of Health Economics* 23(6):1159–1180.

Van Houtven, C., M. Wilson, and E. Clipp. 2005. Informal care intensity and caregiver drug utilization. *Review of Economics of the Household* 3(4):415–433.

Van Houtven, C., E. Z. Oddone, and M. Weinberger. 2010. Informal and formal care infrastructure and perceived need for caregiver training for frail U.S. veterans referred to home and community-based services. *Chronic Illness* 6(1):57–66.

Van Houtven, C., N. B. Coe, and M. M. Skira. 2013. The effect of informal care on work and wages. *Journal of Health Economics* 32(1):240–252.

Wilensky, G. 2018. MA ruling may signal industry readiness to integrate SDH into traditional medical care. *Healthcare Financial Management* 24–25.

Wilson, M., C. H. Van Houtven, S. C. Stearns, and E. C. Clipp. 2007. Depression and missed work among informal caregivers of older individuals with dementia. *Journal of Family and Economic Issues* 28(4):684–698.

Yordi, C. L. 1988. Case management in the social health maintenance organization demonstrations. *Health Care Financing Review* 1988(Suppl):83–88.

Appendix A

Statement of Task

An ad hoc committee will plan and host a 1-day public workshop to examine strategies, approaches, and key challenges to implementation of quality measures for community-based care programs for serious illness.

The workshop will feature invited presentations and panel discussions on topics that may include

- An overview of the role of patient experience and shared decision making in defining quality across a range of evolving care settings, including community-based organizations and home-based care;
- Model programs such as those developed by the BlueCross BlueShield of Massachusetts and the Veterans Health Administration, as well as international efforts such as the Harvard Global Equity Initiative on Pain Control;
- The roles of key stakeholders driving implementation of quality measures, including private and public payers, accreditation organizations, and the National Quality Forum's National Quality Partners;
- Potential tools and mechanisms for implementation, such as public report cards (i.e., Centers for Medicare & Medicaid Services, state-based) and quality improvement efforts undertaken by care programs for serious illness;

- Challenges and opportunities for using potential data sources, including electronic health records, claims, registries, patient-reported data, and crowdsourcing; and
- Ways to develop a feasible approach and timeline for implementing quality measures.

The planning committee will develop the agenda for the workshop, select speakers and discussants, and moderate the discussions. Proceedings of the presentations and the discussions at the workshop will be prepared by a designated rapporteur in accordance with institutional guidelines.

Appendix B

Workshop Agenda

THURSDAY, JULY 19, 2018

8:00 am   **Registration and Breakfast**

8:30 am   **Welcome from the Roundtable on Quality Care for People with Serious Illness**
Leonard D. Schaeffer, University of Southern California (*Chair*)
and
James Tulsky, M.D., Harvard Medical School (*Vice Chair*)

Overview of the Workshop
Joanne Lynn, M.D., Director, Center for Eldercare and Advanced Illness, Altarum, and
Judith R. Peres, LCSW-C, Long-Term and Palliative Care Consultant, Social Work Hospice and Palliative Care Network
Workshop Planning Committee Co-Chairs

8:45 am   **Patient and Family Caregiver Perspective**
Moderator: Judith R. Peres, LCSW-C

MaryAnn, Frank, and Andi Spitale
The Patient and Family Caregiver Experience

9:30 am **Session 1: Framing the Issues of Integrating Health Care and Social Services for People with Serious Illness: Gaps, Challenges, and Opportunities**
Moderator: Lynn Feinberg, M.S.W., Senior Strategic Policy Advisor, AARP Public Policy Institute

Speakers:
—Lauren A. Taylor, M.Div., M.P.H., Doctoral Candidate, Harvard Business School
—Robyn Stone, Senior Vice President of Research, LeadingAge

Panel Discussion/Audience Q&A

10:45 am Break

11:00 am **Session 2: Providing Supportive Services—Exploring the Key Role and Unique Needs of Caregivers**

Moderator: Jeri Miller, Ph.D., National Institute of Nursing Research

Speakers:
—Richard Schulz, Ph.D., Professor of Psychiatry, School of Medicine, Director, University Center for Social and Urban Research, University of Pittsburgh
—Debra Parker Oliver, M.S.W., Ph.D., Professor, University of Missouri Center for Eldercare & Rehabilitation Technology
—Courtney Van Houtven, Ph.D., Research Scientist in Health Services Research and Development in Primary Care, Durham Veterans Affairs and Associate Professor, Duke University Medical Center
—Jennifer L. Wolff, Ph.D., Professor, Johns Hopkins University
—Sarita Gupta, Co-Director, Caring Across Generations

Panel Discussion/Audience Q&A

APPENDIX B 77

12:30 pm   **Lunch and Learn**

E Street Conference Room
Workshop participants pick up lunch and then meet in the E Street Conference Room for information and discussion with organizations involved in providing supportive services.

1:45 pm   **Session 3: Integration of Services—Innovative Partnerships and Collaborations**

Moderator: Peggy Maguire, M.B.A., Senior Vice President, Corporate Accountability and Performance, Cambia Health Foundation

Speakers:
— June Simmons, President and CEO, Partners in Care Foundation
— Gwendolyn Graddy-Dansby, M.D., Chief Medical Officer, Program of All-Inclusive Care for the Elderly (PACE) Southeast Michigan
— Sarah Szanton, Ph.D., ANP, FAAN, Director, Center for Innovative Care in Aging, Johns Hopkins University School of Nursing, Community Aging in Place—Advancing Better Living for Elders (CAPABLE)

Panel Discussion/Audience Q&A

3:15 pm   **Break**

3:30 pm   **Session 4: Policy Challenges and Opportunities for Integrating Health Care and Social Services Nationwide**

Moderator: Joanne Lynn, M.D.

Speakers:
— Kathy Greenlee, J.D., Vice President of Aging & Health Policy, Center for Practical Bioethics
— Bruce Vladeck, Ph.D., Senior Advisor, Greater New York Hospital Association
— Gail Wilensky, Ph.D., Senior Fellow, Project HOPE

Panel Discussion/Audience Q&A

4:30 pm   **Wrap-Up and Adjourn**